NoteS

Clinical Pocket Guide

Darlene D. Pedersen, MSN, APRN, BC

Purchase additional copies of this book
at your health science bookstore or
directly from F. A. Davis by shopping
online at www.fadavis.com or by calling
800-323-3555 (US) or 800-665-1148 (CAN)

A Davis's Notes Book

 F. A. Davis Company • Philadelphia

F. A. Davis Company
1915 Arch Street
Philadelphia, PA 19103

www.fadavis.com

Printed in China by Imago

Last digit indicates print number: 10 9 8 7 6 5 4 3 2

Publisher, Nursing: Robert G. Martone

Project Editor: Tom Ciavarella

Design & Illustration Manager: Joan Wendt

Reviewers: Barbara Bravermann, CRNP, RN, BC; Paulette C. Compton, RN, MSN,
MC; M. Kathryn Corcoran, MSN, CRNP; Brian J. Drew, MSN, APRN, BC; Margie
Eckroth-Bucher, DNSc, RN, APRN, BC; Geraldine D. Greany-Hudson, RN, MS,
APNP/CRNP; Catherine Manuel MacDonald, MN, CNS, APRN-BC; Patricia A. Nutz,
MSN; Dana Olive, MSN, CRNP; Ketan V. Patel, MD; Eula W. Pines, Ph.D, APRN, BC;
Nora Vizzachero, RN, MSN, CRNP; Betty Vreeland, MSN, APRN, NPC, BC; Laurie
Willhite, PharmD, RPh; Robbin Houston Yothers, MSN, CRNP

As new scientific information becomes available through basic and clinical research,
recommended treatments and drug therapies undergo changes. The author(s) and
publisher have done everything possible to make this book accurate, up to date, and
in accord with accepted standards at the time of publication. The author(s), editors,
and publisher are not responsible for errors or omissions or for consequences from
application of the book, and make no warranty, expressed or implied, in regard to the
contents of the book. Any practice described in this book should be applied by the
reader in accordance with professional standards of care used in regard to the
unique circumstances that may apply in each situation. The reader is advised always
to check product information (package inserts) for changes and new information
regarding dose and contraindications before administering any drug. Caution is
especially urged when using new or infrequently ordered drugs.

Place $2\frac{7}{8} \times 2\frac{7}{8}$ **Sticky Notes** here

for a convenient and refillable note pad

✓ **HIPAA Compliant**
✓ **OSHA Compliant**

Waterproof and Reusable
Wipe-Free Pages

Write directly onto any page of *PsychNotes* with a ballpoint pen. Wipe old entries off with an alcohol pad and reuse.

BASICS ASSESS DISORDERS INTERV DRUGS CRISIS GERI TOOLS

Look for our other
Davis's Notes titles

Available Now!

RNotes®: Nurse's Clinical Pocket Guide
ISBN: 0-8036-1060-2

LPN Notes: Nurse's Clinical Pocket Guide
ISBN: 0-8036-1132-3

MedNotes: Nurse's Pharmacology Pocket Guide
ISBN: 0-8036-1109-9

MedSurg Notes: Nurse's Clinical Pocket Guide
ISBN: 0-8036-1115-3

NutriNotes: Nutrition & Diet Therapy Pocket Guide
ISBN: 0-8036-1114-5

IV Therapy Notes: Nurse's Clinical Pocket Guide
ISBN: 0-8036-1288-5

Coming Soon!

LabNotes: Pocket Guide to Lab & Diagnostic Tests
ISBN: 0-8036-1265-6

ECG Notes: Interpretation and Management Pocket Guide
ISBN: 0-8036-1347-4

Mental Health and Mental Illness: Basics

Mental health and mental illness have been defined in many ways but should always be viewed in the context of ethnocultural factors and influence.

Mental Illness/Disorder

The DSM-IV-TR defines **mental illness/disorder** (paraphrased) as: *a clinically significant behavioral or psychological syndrome or pattern associated with distress or disability...with increased risk of death, pain, disability and is not a reasonable (expectable) response to a particular situation.* (APA 2000)

Mental Health

Mental health is defined as: *a state of successful performance of mental function, resulting in productive activities, fulfilling relationships with other people, and the ability to adapt to change and cope with adversity.* (US Surgeon General Report, Dec 1999)

Wellness-illness continuum – Dunn's 1961 text, *High Level Wellness*, altered our concept of health viewing both as on a continuum that was dynamic and changing, focusing on levels of *wellness*. Concepts include: totality, uniqueness, energy, self-integration, energy use, and inner/outer worlds.

Legal Definition of Mental Illness

The **legal definition of insanity/mental illness** applies the M'Naghten Rule, formulated in 1843 and derived from English law. It says that: *a person is innocent by reason of insanity if at the time of committing the act, [the person] was laboring under a defect of reason from disease of the mind as not to know the nature and quality of the act of being done, or if he did not know it, he did not know that what he was doing was wrong.* There are variations of this legal definition by state, and some states have abolished the insanity defense.

Positive Mental Health: Jahoda's Six Major Categories

In 1958, Marie Jahoda developed six major categories of positive mental health:

- Attitudes of individual toward self
- Presence of growth and development, or actualization
- Personality integration
- Autonomy and independence
- Perception of reality, and
- Environmental mastery

The mentally healthy person accepts the self, is self-reliant, and self-confident.

2

Maslow's Hierarchy of Needs

Maslow developed a hierarchy of needs based on attainment of self-actualization, where one becomes highly evolved and attains his or her full potential.

The basic belief is that lower-level needs must be met first in order to advance to the next level of needs. Therefore, physiologic and safety needs must be met before issues related to love and belonging can be addressed, through to self actualization.

SELF-ACTUALIZATION
(The individual possesses a feeling of self-fulfillment and the realization of his or her highest potential.)

SELF-ESTEEM ESTEEM-OF-OTHERS
(The individual seeks self-respect and respect from others, works to achieve success and recognition in work, and desires prestige from accomplishments.)

LOVE AND BELONGING
(Needs are for giving and receiving of affection, companionship, satisfactory interpersonal relationships, and identification with a group.)

SAFETY AND SECURITY
(Needs at this level are for avoiding harm, maintaining comfort, order, structure, physical safety, freedom from fear, and protection.)

PHYSIOLOGICAL NEEDS
(Basic fundamental needs include food, water, air, sleep, exercise, elimination, shelter, and sexual expression.)

General Adaptation Syndrome (Stress-Adaptation Syndrome)

Hans Selye (1976) divided his *stress syndrome* into three stages and, in doing so, pointed out the seriousness of prolonged stress on the body and the need for identification and intervention.

1. **Alarm stage** – This is the immediate physiological (fight or flight) response to a threat or perceived threat.
2. **Resistance** – If the stress continues, the body adapts to the levels of stress and attempts to return to homeostasis.
3. **Exhaustion** – With prolonged exposure and adaptation, the body eventually becomes depleted. There are no more reserves to draw upon, and serious illness may now develop (e.g. hypertension, mental disorders, cancer). Selye teaches us that without intervention, even death is a possibility at this stage.

CLINICAL PEARL: *Identification and treatment of chronic,* posttraumatic stress disorder (PTSD), and unresolved grief, including multiple (compounding) losses, are critical in an attempt to prevent serious illness and improve quality of life.

Fight-or-Flight Response

In the **fight-or-flight response,** if a person is presented with a stressful situation (danger), a physiological (sympathetic nervous system) activates the adrenal glands and cardiovascular system, allowing a person to rapidly adjust to the need to fight or flee a situation.

■ Such physiological response is beneficial in the short term: for instance, in an emergency situation.
■ However, with ongoing, *chronic psychological stressors,* a person continues to experience the same physiological response as if there were a real danger, which eventually physically and emotionally depletes the body.

Theories of Personality Development

Psychoanalytic Theory

Sigmund Freud, who introduced us to the Oedipus complex, hysteria, free association, and dream interpretation, is considered the "Father of Psychiatry." He was concerned with both the *dynamics and structure of the psyche*. He divided the personality into three parts:

■ **Id** – The id developed out of Freud's concept of the pleasure principle. The id comprises primitive, instinctual drives (hunger, sex, aggression). The id says, "I want."

■ **Ego** – It is the ego, or rational mind, that is called upon to control the instinctual impulses of the self-indulgent id. The ego says, "I think/I evaluate."

■ **Superego** – The superego is the conscience of the psyche and monitors the ego. The superego says "I should/I ought." (Hunt 1994)

Topographic Model of the Mind

Freud's topographic model deals with levels of awareness and is divided into three categories:

■ **Unconscious mind** – All mental content and memories *outside of conscious awareness;* becomes conscious through the preconscious mind.

■ **Preconscious mind** – Not within the conscious mind but *can more easily be brought to conscious awareness* (repressive function of instinctual desires or undesirable memories). Reaches consciousness through word linkage.

■ **Conscious mind** – All content and memories *immediately available and within conscious awareness.* Of lesser importance to psychoanalysts.

Key Defense Mechanisms

Defense Mechanism	Example
Denial – Refuses to accept a painful reality, pretending as if it doesn't exist.	A man who snorts cocaine daily, is fired for attendance problems, yet insists he doesn't have a problem.
Displacement – Directing anger toward someone or onto another, less threatening (safer) substitute.	An older employee is publicly embarrassed by a younger boss at work and angrily cuts a driver off on the way home.
Identification – Taking on attributes and characteristics of someone admired.	A young man joins the police academy to become a police-man like his father, whom he respects.
Intellectualization – Excessive focus on logic and reason to avoid the feelings associated with a situation.	An executive who has cancer, requests all studies and blood work, and discusses in detail with her doctor, as if she were speaking about someone else.
Projection – Attributing to others feelings unacceptable to self.	A group therapy client strongly dislikes another member but claims that it is the member who "dislikes her."
Reaction Formation – Expressing an opposite feeling from what is actually felt and is considered undesirable.	John, who despises Jeremy, greets him warmly and offers him food and beverages and special attention.
Sublimation – Redirecting unacceptable feelings or drives into an acceptable channel.	A mother of a child killed in a drive-by shooting becomes involved in legislative change for gun laws and gun violence.
Undoing – Ritualistically negating or undoing intolerable feelings/thoughts.	A man who has thoughts that his father will die must step on sidewalk cracks to prevent this and cannot miss a crack.

Stages of Personality Development

Freud's Psychosexual Development

Age	Stage	Task
0 –18 mo	Oral	Oral gratification
18 mo – 3 yr	Anal	Independence and control (voluntary sphincter control)
3 – 6 yr	Phallic	Genital focus
6 – 12 yr	Latency	Repressed sexuality; channeled sexual drives (sports)
13 – 20 yr	Genital	Puberty with sexual interest in opposite sex

Sullivan's Interpersonal Theory

Age	Stage	Task
0 – 18 mo	Infancy	Anxiety reduction via oral gratification
18 mo – 6 yr	Childhood	Delay in gratification
6 – 9 yr	Juvenile	Satisfying peer relationships
9 – 12 yr	Preadolescence	Satisfying same-sex relationships
12 – 14 yr	Early adolescence	Satisfying opposite-sex relationships
14 – 21 yr	Late adolescence	Lasting intimate opposite-sex relationship

Mahler's Theory of Object Relations

Age	Phase (subphase)	Task
0 – 1 mo	1. Normal autism	Basic needs fulfillment (for survival)
1 – 5 mo	2. Symbiosis 3. Separation – individuation	Awareness of external fulfillment source
5 – 10 mo	– Differentiation	Commencement of separateness from mother figure

Erikson's Psychosocial Theory

Age	Stage	Task
0 – 18 mo	Trust vs mistrust	Basic trust in mother figure & generalizes
18 mo – 3 yr	Autonomy vs shame/doubt	Self control/ independence
3 – 6 yr	Initiative vs guilt	Initiate and direct own activities
6 – 12 yr	Industry vs inferiority	Self confidence through successful performance and recognition
12 – 20 yr	Identity vs role confusion	Task integration from previous stages; secure sense of self
20 – 30 yr	Intimacy vs isolation	Form a lasting relationship or commitment
30 – 65 yr	Generativity vs stagnation	Achieve life's goals; consider future generations
65 yr – death	Ego integrity vs despair	Life review with meaning from both positives and negatives; positive self worth

Age	Phase (subphase)	Task
10 – 16 mo	– *Practicing*	Locomotor independence; awareness of separateness of self
16 – 24 mo	– *Rapprochement*	Acute separateness awareness; seeks emotional refueling from mother figure
24 – 36 mo	– *Consolidation*	Established sense of separateness; internalizes sustained image of loved person/object when out of sight; separation anxiety resolution

Peplau's Interpersonal Theory

Age	Stage	Task
Infant	Depending on others	Learning ways to communicate with primary caregiver for meeting comfort needs
Toddler	Delaying satisfaction	Some delay in self gratification to please others
Early Childhood	Self identification	Acquisition of appropriate roles and behaviors through perception of others' expectations of self
Late Childhood	Participation skills	Competition, compromise, cooperation skills acquisition; sense of one's place in the world

Stages of Personality Development tables modified from Townsend MC. Essentials of Psychiatric Mental Health Nursing, 3rd ed. Philadelphia: FA Davis, 2005, used with permission

Biological Aspects of Mental Illness

- René Descartes (17th C) espoused the theory of the **mind-body dualism (Cartesian dualism)**, wherein the mind (soul) was said to be completely separate from the body.
- Current research and approaches show the connection between mind and body and that newer treatments will develop from a better understanding of both the biological and psychological. (Hunt 1994)
- The US Congress stated that the 1990s would be "The Decade of the Brain," with increased focus and research in the areas of neurobiology, genetics, and biological markers.

Central and Peripheral Nervous System

Central Nervous System

- Brain
  - Forebrain
    - *Cerebrum (frontal, parietal, temporal, and occipital lobes)*
    - *Diencephalon (thalamus, hypothalamus, and limbic system)*
  - *Midbrain*
    - *Mesencephalon*
  - *Hindbrain*
    - *Pons, medulla, and cerebellum*
- Nerve Tissue
  - Neurons
  - Synapses
  - Neurotransmitters
- Spinal Cord
  - Fiber tracts
  - Spinal nerves

Peripheral Nervous System

- Afferent System
  - Sensory neurons (somatic and visceral)

- ■ Efferent System
  - ◆ Somatic nervous system (somatic motor neurons)
  - ◆ Autonomic nervous system
    - • Sympathetic Nervous System
      Visceral motor neurons
    - • Parasympathetic Nervous System
      Visceral motor neurons

The Brain

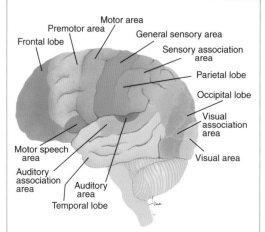

Left cerebral hemisphere showing some of the functional areas that have been mapped. (From Scanlon VC, Sanders T: Essentials of Anatomy and Physiology, ed. 4. FA Davis, Philadelphia 2003, p 170, with permission)

Limbic System

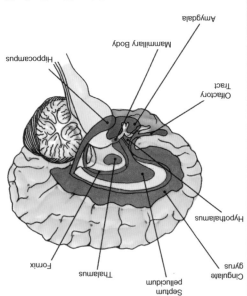

Amygdala

Mammillary Body

Hippocampus

Olfactory Tract

Hypothalamus

Cingulate gyrus

Septum pellucidum

Thalamus

Fornix

The limbic system and its structures (Adapted from Scanlon VC, Sanders T: Essentials of Anatomy and Physiology, ed. 4. FA Davis, Philadelphia 2003, with permission)

Autonomic Nervous System

Sympathetic and Parasympathetic Effects

Structure	Sympathetic	Parasympathetic
Eye (pupil)	Dilation	Constriction
Nasal Mucosa	Mucus reduction	Mucus increased
Salivary Gland	Saliva reduction	Saliva increased
Heart	Rate increased	Rate decreased
Arteries	Constriction	Dilation
Lung	Bronchial muscle relaxation	Bronchial muscle contraction
Gastrointestinal Tract	Decreased motility	Increased motility
Liver	Conversion of glycogen to glucose increased	Glycogen synthesis
Kidney	Decreased urine	Increased urine
Bladder	Contraction of sphincter	Relaxation of sphincter
Sweat Glands	↑Sweating	No change

Autonomic Nervous System (continued)

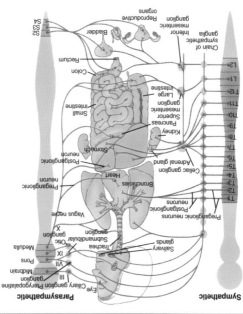

Parasympathetic

Eye — Ciliary ganglion — Pterygopalatine ganglion
III
Midbrain
Pons — VII
Medulla — IX
X
Submandibular ganglion
Otic ganglion
Salivary — Trachea
Vagus nerve
Bronchioles
Heart
Preganglionic neuron
Postganglionic neuron
Stomach
Small intestine
Large intestine
Colon
Rectum
Bladder
Reproductive organs
SS2
SS3
SS4

Sympathetic

Pancreas
Kidney
Adrenal gland
Celiac ganglion
Superior mesenteric ganglion
Inferior mesenteric ganglion
Chain of sympathetic ganglia
Preganglionic neurons
Postganglionic neurons
T1 T2 T3 T4 T5 T6 T7 T8 T9 T10 T11 T12 L1 L2

The sympathetic system is shown on the left and the parasympathetic system is shown on the right (the divisions are bilateral). (From Scanlon VC, Sanders T: Essentials of Anatomy and Physiology, ed. 4. FA Davis, Philadelphia 2003, p 180, with permission)

14

Synapse Transmission

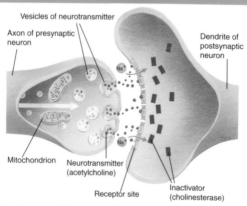

Vesicles of neurotransmitter

Axon of presynaptic neuron

Dendrite of postsynaptic neuron

Mitochondrion

Neurotransmitter (acetylcholine)

Receptor site

Inactivator (cholinesterase)

Impulse transmission at a synapse. Arrow indicates direction of electrical impulse. (From Scanlon VC, Sanders T: Essentials of Anatomy and Physiology, ed. 4. FA Davis, Philadelphia 2003, p 159, with permission)

Neurotransmitters

Neurotransmitter Functions and Effects

Neurotransmitter	Function	Effect
Dopamine	Inhibitory	Fine movement, emotional behavior. Implicated in schizophrenia and Parkinson's.
Serotonin	Inhibitory	Sleep, mood, eating behavior. Implicated in mood disorders, anxiety, and violence.
Norepinephrine	Excitatory	Arousal, wakefulness, learning. Implicated in anxiety and addiction.
Gamma-aminobutyric acid (GABA)	Inhibitory	Anxiety states.
Acetylcholine	Excitatory	Arousal, attention, movement. Increase = spasms and decrease = paralysis.

Legal-Ethical Issues

Confidentiality

Confidentiality in all of health care is important but notably so in psychiatry because of possible discriminatory treatment of those with mental illness. All individuals have a right to privacy, and all client records and communications should be kept confidential.

Dos and Don'ts of Confidentiality

■ Do not discuss clients by using their actual names or any identifier that could be linked to a particular client (e.g., name/date of birth on an X-ray/assessment form).

- Be sensitive to the rights of clients and their right to confidentiality.
- Do not discuss client particulars outside of a private, professional environment. Do not discuss with family members or friends.
- Be particularly careful in elevators of hospitals or community centers. You never know who might be on the elevator with you.
- Even in educational presentations, protect client identity by changing names (John Doe) and obtaining all (informed consent) permissions.
- Every client has the right to confidential and respectful treatment.
- Accurate, objective record keeping is important, and documentation is significant legally in demonstrating what was actually done for client care. If not documented, treatments are not considered done.

When Confidentiality Must Be Breached

- **Confidentiality and Child Abuse** – If it is suspected or clear that a child is being abused or in danger of abuse (physical/sexual/emotional) or neglect, the health professional must report such abuse as mandated by the Child Abuse Prevention Treatment Act, originally enacted in 1974 (PL 93–247).
- **Confidentiality and Elder Abuse** – If suspected or clear that an elder is being abused or in danger of abuse or neglect, then the health professional must also report this abuse.
- **Tarasoff Principle/Duty to Warn** (Tarasoff v. Regents of the University of California 1976) – Refers to the responsibility of a therapist, health professional, or nurse to warn a potential victim of imminent danger (a threat to harm person) and breach confidentiality. The person in danger and others (able to protect person) must be notified of the intended harm.

The Health Insurance Portability and Accountability (HIPAA) Act (1996)

Enacted on August 21, 1996, HIPAA was established with the goal of assuring that an individual's health information is properly protected while allowing the flow of health information. (HIPAA, 2004; US Department of Health and Human Services, 2004)

Types of Commitment

- **Voluntary** – An individual decides treatment is needed and admits him/herself to a hospital, leaving of own volition – unless a professional (psychiatrist/other professional) decides that the person is a danger to him/herself or others.

- **Involuntary** – Involuntary commitments include: 1) emergency commitments, including those unable to meet the basic personal needs; and 2) involuntary outpatient commitment (IOC).

  - ◆ **Emergency** – Involves *imminent* danger to self or others; has demonstrated a *clear and present danger to self or others*. Usually initiated by health professionals, authorities, and sometimes friends or family. Person is threatening to harm self or others. Or evidence that the person is unable to care for her- or himself (nourishment, personal, medical, safety) with reasonable probability that death will result within a month.

  - ◆ **302 Emergency Involuntary Commitment** – If a person is an immediate danger to self or others or is *in danger* due to a lack of ability to care for self, then an emergency psychiatric evaluation may be filed (section 302). This person must then be evaluated by a psychiatrist and released, or psychiatrist must then uphold petition (patient admitted for up to five days).

(Laben & Crofts 1998; emergency commitments 2004)

Restraints and Seclusion – Behavioral Healthcare

The Joint Commission on Accreditation of Healthcare Organizations (JCAHO) wants to reduce the use of behavioral restraints but has set forth guidelines for safety in the event they are used.

- ■ In an emergency situation, restraints may be applied by an authorized and qualified nonlicensed independent practitioner staff member.

- ■ Following application of restraints, the following time frames must be adhered to for reevaluation/reordering:

  - ◆ Within first hour, physician or licensed independent practitioner (LIP) must evaluate the patient, after application of restraint.

- After the first 4-hour order expires, a qualified RN or other authorized staff person reevaluates individual and need to continue restraint/seclusion.
- If restraint/seclusion still needed – LIP notified and order (written/verbal) given for 4 hours.
- After 8 hours in restraint/seclusion – evaluation of continued need by LIP is done face to face. If needed, another 4 hours is ordered (written).
- Four-hour RN or other qualified staff reassessment and 8-hour face-to-face evaluation repeated, as long as restraint and seclusion are clinically necessary. (JCAHO 2004)

■ The *American Psychiatric Nurses Association* and *International Society of Psychiatric-Mental Health Nurses* are committed to the *reduction of seclusion and restraint* and have developed position statements, with a vision of eventually eliminating seclusion and restraint. (APNA 2004; ISPN 2004)

ALERT: Restraint of a patient may be both physical or pharmacological (chemical) and infringes on a patient's freedom of movement and may result in injury (physical or psychological) and/or death. Such use cannot be taken lightly. There has been a movement – for many substantiated reasons – toward *restraint reduction*. There must be an evaluation based on benefit: risk consideration and a leaning toward alternative solutions. Restraints need to be a last resort (Omnibus Budget Reconciliation Act of 1987 [nursing homes]). Restraints may be used when there is dangerous behavior and to protect the patient and others. You need to become familiar with the standards as set forth by JCAHO and any state regulations and hospital policies. *The least restrictive method should be used and considered first, before using more restrictive interventions.*

A Patient's Bill of Rights
■ First adopted in 1973 by the American Hospital Association, *A Patient's Bill of Rights* was revised on October 21, 1992
■ Sets forth an expectation of treatment and care that will allow for improved collaboration between patients, health care providers, and institutions resulting in better patient care. (American Hospital Association 2004)

Informed Consent

■ Every adult person has the right to decide what can and cannot be done to his or her own body (Schloendorff v. Society of New York Hospital, 105 NE 92 [NY 1914]).

■ Assumes a person is capable of making an informed decision about own health care.

■ State regulations vary, but mental illness does not mean that a person is or should be assumed incapable of making decisions related to his or her own care.

Patients have a right to:
  ♦ Information about their treatment and any procedures to be performed
  ♦ Know the inherent risks and benefits

■ Without this information (specific information, risks, and benefits) a person cannot make an informed decision. The above also holds true for those who might participate in research. (Laben & Crofts Yorker 1998)

Right to Refuse Treatment/Medication

■ Just as a person has the right to accept treatment, he or she also has the right to refuse treatment to the extent permitted *by the law and to be informed of the medical consequences of his actions.*

■ In some emergency situations, a patient can be medicated or treated against his/her will, but state laws vary and so it is imperative to become knowledgeable about applicable state laws. (American Hospital Association 2004; Laben & Crofts Yorker 1998)

Psychiatric Assessment

Psychiatric History and Assessment Tool

Identifying/Demographic Information

Name	Room No.
Primary Care Provider:	
DOB	Age Sex
Race:	Ethnicity:
Marital Status:	No. Marriages:
If married/divorced/separated/ widowed, how long?	
Occupation/School (grade):	
Highest Education Level:	
Religious Affiliation:	
City of Residence:	
Name/Phone # of Significant Other:	
Primary Language Spoken:	
Accompanied by:	
Admitted from:	
Previous Psychiatric Hospitalizations (#):	
Chief Complaint (in patient's own words):	
DSM-IV Diagnosis (previous/current):	
Nursing Diagnosis:	

Family Members/Significant Others Living in Home			
Name	Relationship	Age	Occupation/Grade

Family Members/Significant Others Not in Home			
Name	Relationship	Age	Occupation/Grade

Children		
Name	Age	Living at Home?

CLINICAL PEARL: Compare what the client says with what other family members, friends, or significant others say about situations or previous treatments. It is usually helpful to gather information from those who have observed/lived with the client and can provide *another valuable source/side of information*. The *reliability of the client* in recounting the past must be considered and should be noted.

Genogram - See *Intervention Tab* for sample genogram and common genogram symbols.

Past Psychiatric Treatments/Medications

It is important to obtain a history of any previous psychiatric hospitalizations, the number of hospitalizations and dates, and to record all current/past psychotropic medications, as well as other medications the client may be taking. Ask the client what has worked in the past, and also what has *not worked*, for both treatments and medications.

Inpatient Treatment

Facility/Location	Dates From/To	Diagnosis	Treatments	Response(s)

Outpatient Treatments/Services

Psychiatrist/Therapist	Location	Diagnosis	Treatment	Response(s)

Psychotropic Medications (Previous Treatments)

Name	Dose/Dosages	Treatment Length	Response	Comments

Current Psychotropic Medications/Other Medications

Current Psychotropic Medications

Name	Dose/Dosages	Date Started	Response(s)	Serum Levels

Other Current Medications, Herbals, and OTC Medications

Name	Dose/Dosages	Date Started	Response(s)	Comments

CLINICAL PEARL: It is important to ask about any herbals, OTC medications (e.g., pseudoephedrine), or nontraditional treatments as client may not think to mention these when questioned about current medications. *Important herbals include, but are not limited to:* St. John's wort, ephedra (ma huang), ginseng, kava kava, and yohimbe. These can interact with psychotropics or other medications or cause anxiety and/or drowsiness, as well as other adverse physiological reactions. Be sure to record and then report any additional or herbal medications to the psychiatrist, advanced practice nurse, psychiatric nurse, and professional team staff.

Medical History (*See Clinical Pearls for Italics*)

TPR:	BP:
Height:	Weight:

Cardiovascular (CV)
Does client have or ever had the following disorders/symptoms (include date):

Hypertension	Murmurs	Chest Pain (Angina)
Palpitations/ Tachycardia	Shortness of Breath	Ankle Edema/Congestive Heart Failure
Fainting/Syncope	Myocardial Infarction	High Cholesterol
Leg Pain (Claudication)	*Arrhythmias*	*Other CV Disease*
Heart Bypass	Angioplasty	Other CV surgery

CLINICAL PEARL: Heterocyclic antidepressants must be used with caution with *cardiovascular disease*. TCAs may produce life-threatening *arrhythmias* and ECG changes.

Central Nervous System (CNS)

Headache	Head Injury	Tremors
Dizziness/Vertigo	Loss of Consciousness (LOC); how long?	Stroke
Myasthenia Gravis	Parkinson's Disease	Dementia
Brain Tumor	Seizure Disorder	Multiple Sclerosis
TIAs	Other	Surgeries

CLINICAL PEARL: Remember that *myasthenia gravis* is a contraindication to the use of antipsychotics; *tremors* could be due to a disease such as *Parkinson's* or could be a side effect of a psychotropic (lithium/antipsychotic). Sometimes the elderly may be diagnosed as having *dementia* when in fact they are depressed (pseudodementia). Use TCAs cautiously with *seizure disorders*; buproprion use contraindicated in seizure disorder.

Dermatological/Skin

Does client have or ever had the following disorders/symptoms (include date):

Psoriasis	Hair Loss	Itching
Rashes	Acne	Other/Surgeries

CLINICAL PEARL: Lithium can precipitate psoriasis or psoriatic *arthritis* in patients with a history of psoriasis, or the psoriasis may be new onset. *Acne* is also a possible reaction to lithium (new onset or exacerbation) and lithium may result in, although rarely, *hair loss (alopecia)*. *Rashes* in patients on carbamaze-pine or lamotrigine may be a sign of a life-threatening muco-cutaneous reaction, such as Stevens-Johnson syndrome (SJS). Discontinue medication/immediate medical attention needed.

Endocrinology/Metabolic

Does client have or ever had the following disorders/symptoms (include date):

Polydipsia	Polyuria	*Diabetes Type 1 or 2*
Hyperthyroidism	*Hypothyroidism*	Hirsutism
PCOS	Other	Surgeries

CLINICAL PEARL: Clients on lithium should be observed and tested for *hypothyroidism*. Atypical and older antipsychotics are associated with *new-onset diabetes (need periodic testing: FBS, HgbA1c, lipids; BMI, etc).*

Eye, Ears, Nose, Throat

Does client have or ever had the following disorders/symptoms (include date):

Eye Pain	Halo around Light Source	*Blurring*
Red eye	Double vision	Flashing Lights/Floaters
Glaucoma	Tinnitus	Ear Pain/Otitis Media
Hoarseness	Other	Other/Surgeries

CLINICAL PEARL: *Eye pain and halo around a light source* are possible symptoms of glaucoma. *Closed-angle glaucoma* is a true *emergency* and requires immediate medical attention to prevent blindness. Anticholinergics (low-potency antipsychotics [chlorpromazine] or tricyclics) can cause *blurred vision.* Check for *history of glaucoma* as antipsychotics are contraindicated.

Gastrointestinal
Does client have or ever had the following disorders/symptoms (include date):

Nausea & Vomiting	Diarrhea	Constipation
GERD	Crohn's Disease	Colitis
Colon Cancer	Irritable Bowel Syndrome	Other/Surgeries

CLINICAL PEARL: *Nausea* is a common side effect of many medications; tricyclic antidepressants can cause *constipation*. Nausea seems to be more common with paroxetine. Over time clients adjust to these side effects, and so no decision should be made about effectiveness/side effects or changing medications without a reasonable trial.

Genito-urinary/Reproductive
Does client have or ever had the following disorders/symptoms (include date):

Miscarriages? Y/N		Abortions? Y/N	
# When?		# When?	

Nipple Discharge	Amenorrhea	Gynecomastia
Lactation	Dysuria	Urinary Incontinence
Pregnancy Problems	Postpartum Depression	Sexual Dysfunction
Prostate Problems	Menopause	Fibrocystic Disease
Penile Discharge	UTI	Pelvic Pain

| Renal Disease | Urinary Cancer | Breast Cancer |
| Other/Surgeries | Other Gynecologic Cancer | Other |

CLINICAL PEARL: Antipsychotics have an effect on the endocrinologic system by affecting the tuberoinfundibular system. Those on antipsychotics may experience *gynecomastia and lactation (men also)*. Women may experience *amenorrhea*. Some drugs (TCAs), such as amitriptyline, must be used with caution with BPH.

Respiratory

Does client have or ever had (include date):

Chronic Cough	Sore Throat	Bronchitis
Asthma	COPD	Pneumonia
Cancer (Lung/Throat)	Sleep Apnea	Other/Surgeries

Other Questions:

Allergies (food/environmental/pet/contact)

Diet _____

_____

Drug Allergies _____

_____

Accidents _____

_____

High Prolonged Fever _____

Tobacco Use _____

Childhood Illnesses _____

Fractures _____

Menses Began _____
Birth Control _____
Disabilities (hearing/speech/movement) _____
Pain (describe/location/length of time [over or under 3 months]/severity between 1 [least] and 10 [worst])/Treatment

Family History

Mental Illness _____

Medical Disorders _____

Substance Abuse _____

Please note who in the family has the problem/disorder.

Substance Use
Prescribed Drugs

Name	Dosage	Reason

Street Drugs

Name	Amount/Day	Reason

Alcohol

Name	Amount/Day/Week	Reason

Substance History and Assessment Tool

1. When you were growing up, did anyone in your family use substances (alcohol or drugs)? If yes, how did the substance use affect the family?

2. When (how old) did you use your first substance (e.g., alcohol, cannabis) and what was it?

3. How long have you been using a substance(s) regularly? Weeks, months, years?

4. Pattern of abuse
   a. When do you use substances?
   b. How much and how often do you use?
   c. Where are you when you use substances and with whom?

5. When did you last use; what was it and how much did you use?

6. Has substance use caused you any problems with family, friends, job, school, the legal system, other? If yes, describe:

7. Have you ever had an injury or accident because of substance abuse? If yes, describe:

8. Have you ever been arrested for a DUI because of your drinking or other substance use?

9. Have you ever been arrested or placed in jail because of drugs or alcohol?

10. Have you ever experienced memory loss the morning after substance use (can't remember what you did the night before)? Describe the event and feelings about the situation:

11. Have you ever tried to stop your substance use? If yes, why were you not able to stop? Did you have any physical symptoms such as shakiness, sweating, nausea, headaches, insomnia, or seizures?

12. Describe a typical day in your life.

13. Are there any changes you would like to make in your life? If so, describe:

14. What plans or ideas do you have for making these changes?

15. History of withdrawal:

Other comments:

Modified from Townsend MC. Psychiatric Mental Health Nursing: Concepts of Care, 4th ed. Philadelphia: FA Davis, 2003, with permission

● ● ● ● ● ● ● ● ● ● ●

35

CAGE Screening Questionnaire

(C) Have you ever felt the need to <u>Cut Down</u> on your drinking/ use of drugs? Y__ N__

(A) Have you been <u>Annoyed</u> by the criticism of others about your drinking/drug use? Y__ N__

(G) Have you felt <u>Guilty</u> about the amount of drinking you do? Y__ N__

(E) Have you ever had an <u>Eye Opener</u> (drink) first thing in the morning, to steady your nerves? Y__ N__

A positive (yes) response to two or more questions suggests that there is an alcohol/substance abuse problem.
(Ewing JA: Detecting alcoholism: The CAGE questionnaire. JAMA 252:1905–1907, 1984.)

Note: The need to <u>cut down</u> is related to tolerance (needing more substance for same effect) and the <u>eye opener</u> is related to withdrawal syndrome (reduction/cessation of substance).

Short Michigan Alcohol Screening Test (SMAST)

■ Do you feel you are a normal drinker? [no] Y__ N__
■ Does someone close to you worry about your drinking? [yes] Y__ N__
■ Do you feel guilty about your drinking? [yes] Y__ N__
■ Do friends/relatives think you're a normal drinker? [no] Y__ N__
■ Can you stop drinking when you want to? [no] Y__ N__
■ Have you ever attended an AA meeting? [yes] Y__ N__
■ Has drinking created problems between you and a loved one/relative? [yes] Y__ N__
■ Gotten in trouble at work because of drinking? [yes] Y__ N__
■ Neglected obligations/family/work 2 days in a row because of drinking? [yes] Y__ N__
■ Gone to anyone for help for your drinking? [yes] Y__ N__
■ Ever been in a hospital because of drinking? [yes] Y__ N__
■ Arrested for drunk driving or DUI? [yes] Y__ N__
■ Arrested for other drunken behavior? [yes] Y__ N__   Total =

Five or more positive items suggests alcohol problem.
(Positive answers are in brackets above) (Selzer 1975)

Reprinted with permission *from Journal of Studies on Alcohol,* vol. 36, pp. 117–126, 1975. Copyright by Journal of Studies on Alcohol, Inc., Rutgers Center of Alcohol Studies, Piscataway, NJ 08854

Mental Status Assessment and Tool

The components of the mental status assessment are:

- General Appearance
- Behavior/Activity
- Speech and Language
- Mood and Affect
- Thought Process and Content
- Perceptual Disturbances
- Memory/Cognitive
- Judgment and Insight

Each component must be approached in a methodical manner so that a thorough evaluation of the client can be done from a mood, thought, appearance, insight, judgment, and overall perspective.

It is important to document all these findings even though this record represents one point in time. It is helpful over time to see any patterns (regressions/improvement) and to gain an understanding of any changes that would trigger a need to reevaluate the client or suggest a decline in functioning.

Mental Status Assessment Tool

Identifying Information

Name	Age
Sex	Race/Ethnicity
Significant Other	Educational Level
Religion	Occupation

Presenting problem:

Appearance

Grooming/dress

Hygiene

Eye contact

Posture _____

Identifying features (marks/scars/tattoos) _____

Appearance versus stated age _____

Overall appearance _____

CLINICAL PEARL: It is helpful to ask the client to talk about him/herself and to *ask open-ended questions* to help the client express thoughts and feelings; e.g., "Tell me why you are here?" Encourage further discussion with: "Tell me more." A less direct and more conversational tone at the beginning of the interview may help reduce the client's anxiety and set the stage for the trust needed in a therapeutic relationship.

Behavior/Activity (check if present)

Hyperactive _____

Agitated _____

Psychomotor retardation _____

Calm _____

Tremors _____

Tics _____

Unusual movements/gestures _____

Catatonia _____

Akathisia _____

Rigidity _____

Facial movements (jaw/lip smacking) _____

Other _____

Speech

Slow/rapid _____

Pressured _____

Tone _____

Volume (loud/soft) _____

Fluency (mute/hesitation/latency of response) _____

Attitude

Is client:

Cooperative _____ Uncooperative _____

Distant _____ Warm/friendly _____

Suspicious _____ Guarded _____

Combative _____ Aggressive _____

Hostile _____ Aloof _____

Apathetic _____ Other _____

Mood and Affect

Is client:

Depressed _____ Sad _____ Elated _____

Irritable _____

Anxious _____

Guilty _____ Fearful _____

Worried _____

Angry _____

Hopeless _____ Labile _____

Mixed (anxious and depressed) _____

Is Client's Affect:

Flat _____

Blunted or diminished _____

Appropriate _____

Inappropriate/incongruent (sad and smiling/laughing) _____

Other _____

Thought Process

Concrete thinking _____

Circumstantiality _____

Tangentiality _____

Loose association _____

Echolalia _____

Flight of ideas _____

Perseveration _____

Clang associations _____

Blocking _____

Word salad _____

Derailment _____

Other: _____

Thought Content
Does client have:
Delusions (grandiose/persecution/reference/somatic):
_____
Suicidal/homicidal thoughts _____
If homicidal, toward whom? _____
Obsessions _____
Paranoia _____
Phobias _____
Magical thinking _____
Poverty of speech _____
Other _____

CLINICAL PEARL: Questions around suicide and homicide need
to be direct. For instance, *Are you thinking of harming yourself/
another person right now?* (If another, who?) Clients will
usually admit to suicidal thoughts *if asked directly* but will not
always volunteer this information. Any threat to harm someone
else requires informing the potential victim and the authorities.
(*See When Confidentiality Must be Breached, Tarasoff
Principle/Duty to Warn,* in Basics Tab.)

Perceptual Disturbances
Is client experiencing:
Visual Hallucinations _____
Auditory Hallucinations _____
    Commenting _____
    Discussing _____
    Commanding _____
    Loud _____
    Soft _____
    Other _____
Other Hallucination (olfactory/tactile) _____
Illusions _____
Depersonalization _____
Other _____

Memory/Cognitive
Orientation (time/place/person)

Memory (recent/remote/confabulation)

Level of alertness

Insight and Judgment

Insight (awareness of the nature of the illness)

Judgment

"What would you do if you saw a fire in a movie theater?" "How will you manage financially once you leave the hospital?"

Other

Impulse control

Other

DSM-IV-TR Multiaxial Classification and Tool

Allows for assessment on various axes, which provides information on different domains, and assists in planning interventions and identifying outcomes. Includes GAF (axis V) (explained later).

Components

Axis I: Clinical Disorder (or focus of clinical attention)
Axis II: Personality Disorders/Mental Retardation
Axis III: General Medical Conditions
Axis IV: Psychosocial/Environmental
Axis V: Global Assessment of Functioning (GAF)
  Current:
  Past Year, highest level:
  Admission:
  Discharge:

Sample DSM-IV-TR Multiaxial Classifications

Axis I: V61.10 Partner Relational Problem
Axis II: 301.6 Dependent Personality Disorder
Axis III: 564.1 Irritable Bowel Syndrome
Axis IV: Two small daughters at home
Axis V: GAF (current) 65
  Past year, highest level: 80

Axis I: 296.44 Bipolar I Disorder, most recent episode manic,
  severe with psychotic features
Axis II: 301.83 Borderline Personality Disorder
Axis III: 704.00 Alopecia
Axis IV: Unemployed
Axis V: GAF Admission: 28
Discharge: 62

DSM-IV-TR Multiaxial Evaluation Tool*

Axis I:
Clinical Disorder/Clinical Focus
Include diagnostic code/
DSM-IV name

Axis II:
Personality Disorders/
Mental Retardation; *include*
Diagnostic code/DSM-IV name

Axis III:
Any General Medical Conditions
Include ICD-9-CM codes/names

Axis IV:
Psychosocial/
Environmental Problems:
(family/primary support group/
social/occupational/educational/
health care/legal/crime/other)

Axis V (**GAF**):
Current/hospital:
Highest level past year/discharge:

---

*See *Tools Tab* for DSM-IV-TR Classification/Codes

Multiaxial form reprinted with permission from the Diagnostic
  and Statistical Manual of Mental Disorders, Fourth Edition, Text
  Revision (Copyright 2000). American Psychiatric Association.

CLINICAL PEARL: It is often an Axis I disorder (depression/anxiety) that brings a client into therapy but an Axis II disorder (dependent/borderline personality) that keeps the client in therapy. Problems/crises continue in spite of treatment.

Global Assessment of Functioning (GAF)/Scale

The GAF provides an *overall* rating of assessment of function. It is concerned with psychosocial/occupational aspects and divided into ten ranges of functioning, covering both *symptom severity and functioning*. The GAF is recorded as a numerical value on Axis V of the Multiaxial System (see above).

Global Assessment of Functioning (GAF) Scale

Code	Note: Use intermediate codes when appropriate (e.g., 45, 68, 72).
100 91	Superior functioning in a wide range of activities, life's problems never seem to get out of hand, sought out by others because of his or her many positive qualities. No symptoms.
90 81	Absent or minimal symptoms (e.g., mild anxiety before an exam), good functioning in all areas, interested and involved in a wide range of activities, socially effective; generally satisfied with life; no more than general problems or concerns (e.g., an occasional argument with family members).
80 71	If symptoms are present, they are transient and expectable reactions to psychosocial stressors (e.g., difficulty concentrating after family argument); slight impairment in social, work, or school functioning (e.g., temporarily falling behind in schoolwork).
70 61	Some mild symptoms (e.g., depressed mood and mild insomnia) OR some difficulty in social, occupational, or school functioning (e.g., occasional truancy, or theft within the household), but generally functioning pretty well, has some meaningful interpersonal relationships.

Code	
60 51	Moderate symptoms (e.g., flat affect and circumstantial speech, occasional panic attacks) OR moderate difficulty in social, occupational, or school functioning (e.g., few friends, conflicts with peers or co-workers).
50 41	Serious symptoms (e.g., suicidal ideation, severe obsessional rituals, frequent shoplifting) OR serious impairment in social, occupational, or school functioning (e.g., no friends, unable to keep a job).
40 31	Some impairment in reality testing or communication (e.g., speech is at times illogical, obscure, or irrelevant) OR major impairment in several areas, such as work, school, family relations, judgment, thinking, or mood (e.g., depressed man avoids friends, neglects family, and is unable to work; child frequently beats up younger children, is defiant at home, and is failing at school).
30 21	Behavior is considerably influenced by delusions or hallucinations OR serious impairment in communication or judgment (e.g., sometimes incoherent, acts grossly inappropriately, suicidal preoccupation) OR inability to function in almost all areas (e.g., stays in bed all day; no job, home, or friends).
20 11	Some danger of hurting self or others (e.g., suicide attempts without clear expectation of death; frequently violent; manic excitement) OR occasionally fails to maintain minimal personal hygiene (e.g., smears feces) OR gross impairment in communication (e.g., largely incoherent or mute).
10 1	Persistent danger of severely hurting self or others (e.g., recurrent violence) OR persistent inability to maintain minimal personal hygiene OR serious suicidal act with clear expectation of death.

0 = Inadequate information
GAF scale reprinted with permission from the Diagnostic and Statistical Manual of Mental Disorders, Fourth Edition, Text Revision (Copyright 2000). American Psychiatric Association.

Abnormal Involuntary Movement Scale (AIMS)

AIMS is a five- to ten-minute clinician/other trained rater (psychiatric nurse) scale to assess for tardive dyskinesia. AIMS is not a scored scale but rather a *comparative scale* documenting changes over time (Guy 1976).

- Baseline should be done before instituting pharmacotherapy and then every three (3) to six (6) months thereafter. Check with Federal and hospital regulations for time frames. Long-term care facilities are required to perform the AIMS at initiation of antipsychotic therapy and every six months thereafter.

AIMS Examination Procedure

Either before or after completing the examination procedure, observe the client unobtrusively, at rest (e.g., in waiting room). The chair to be used in the examination should be hard and firm without arms.

- Ask client to remove shoes and socks.
- Ask client if there is anything in his/her mouth (e.g., gum, candy); if there is, to remove it.
- Ask client about the *current* condition of his/her teeth. Ask client if he/she wears dentures. Do teeth or dentures bother the client *now?*
- Ask client whether he/she notices any movements in mouth, face, hands, or feet. If yes, ask to describe and to what extent they *currently* bother client or interfere with his/her activities.
- Have client sit in chair with hands on knees, legs slightly apart and feet flat on floor. (Look at entire body for movements while client is in this position.)
- Ask client to sit with hands hanging unsupported; if male, between legs; if female and wearing a dress, hanging over knees. (Observe hands and other body areas.)
- Ask client to open mouth. (Observe tongue at rest in mouth.) Do this twice.
- Ask client to protrude tongue. (Observe abnormalities of tongue movement.) Do this twice.
- Ask client to tap thumb, with each finger, as rapidly as possible for 10 to 15 seconds; separately with right hand, then with left hand. (Observe facial and leg movements.)
- Flex and extend client's left and right arms (one at a time). (Note any rigidity.)

AIMS Examination Procedure *(Continued)*
- Ask client to stand up. (Observe in profile. Observe all body areas again, hips included.)
- Ask client to extend both arms outstretched in front with palms down. (Observe trunk, legs, and mouth.)
- Have client walk a few paces, turn, and walk back to chair. (Observe hands and gait.) Do this twice.

AIMS Rating Form

Name		Rater Name	
Date		ID #	

Instructions: Complete the above examination procedure before making ratings. For movement ratings, circle the highest severity observed.	Code: 0: None 1: Minimal, may be extreme normal 2: Mild 3: Moderate 4: Severe

Facial and Oral Movements	**1. Muscles of Facial Expression** • e.g., Movements of forehead, eyebrows, periorbital area, cheeks • Include frowning, blinking, smiling, and grimacing.	0 1 2 3 4
	2. Lips and Perioral Area e.g., puckering, pouting, smacking	0 1 2 3 4
	3. Jaw e.g., biting, clenching, chewing, mouth opening, lateral movement	0 1 2 3 4
	4. Tongue Rate only increase in movements both in and out of mouth, NOT the inability to sustain movement.	0 1 2 3 4

(Continued on following page)

Extremity Movements	**5. Upper** *(arms, wrists, hands, fingers)* • Include choreic movements (i.e., rapid, objectively purposeless, irregular, spontaneous), athetoid movements (i.e., slow, irregular, complex, serpentine). • Do NOT include tremor (i.e., repetitive, regular, rhythmic).	0 1 2 3 4
	6. Lower *(legs, knees, ankles, toes)* e.g., lateral knee movement, foot tapping, heel dropping, foot squirming, inversion and eversion of the foot	0 1 2 3 4
Trunk Movements	**7. Neck, shoulders, hips** e.g., rocking, twisting, squirming, pelvic gyrations	0 1 2 3 4
Global Judgments	**8. Severity of Abnormal Movements**	0 1 2 3 4
	9. Incapacitation Due to Abnormal Movements	0 1 2 3 4
	10. Client's Awareness of Abnormal Movements Rate only client's report.	0 1 2 3 4
Dental Status	**11. Current Problems with Teeth and/or Dentures**	0: No 1: Yes
	12. Does Client Usually Wear Dentures?	0: No 1: Yes

(Continued)

Geriatric Depression Rating Scale (GDS)

Short Version

Choose the best answer for how you have felt *over the past week* (circle yes or no):

1. Are you basically satisfied with your life? YES/**NO**
2. Have you dropped many of your activities and interests? **YES**/NO
3. Do you feel that your life is empty? **YES**/NO
4. Do you often get bored? **YES**/NO
5. Are you in good spirits most of the time? YES/**NO**
6. Are you afraid that something bad is going to happen to you? **YES**/NO
7. Do you feel happy most of the time? YES/**NO**
8. Do you often feel helpless? **YES**/NO
9. Do you prefer to stay at home, rather than going out and doing new things? **YES**/NO
10. Do you feel you have more problems with memory than most? **YES**/NO
11. Do you think it is wonderful to be alive now? YES/**NO**
12. Do you feel pretty worthless the way you are now? **YES**/NO
13. Do you feel full of energy? YES/**NO**
14. Do you feel that your situation is hopeless? **YES**/NO
15. Do you think that most people are better off than you are? **YES**/NO   Total Score =

Bold answers = depression.

GDS Scoring:

12–15   Severe depression
8–11   Moderate depression
5–8   Mild depression
0–4   Normal
(Yesavage et al. 1983; Sheikh 1986)
GDS website: http://www.stanford.edu/~yesavage/

ALERT: As with all rating scales, further evaluation and monitoring are often needed. Be sure to perform a Mini-Mental State Examination (MMSE) first to screen for/rule out dementia (cognitive deficits).

Mini-Mental State Examination (MMSE)

The *Mini-Mental State Examination* is a brief (10-minute) standardized, reliable screening instrument used to screen for cognitive impairment and commonly used to screen for dementia. It evaluates orientation, registration, concentration, language, short-term memory, and visual-spatial aspects and can be scored quickly (24 - 30 = normal; 18 - 23 = mild/moderate cognitive impairment; 0 - 17 = severe cognitive impairment). (Folstein et al. 1975; Psychological Assessment Resources, Inc.)

The Clock-Drawing Test

Another test that is said to be possibly more sensitive to *early* dementia is the clock-drawing test. There are many variations and clock is first drawn (by clinician) and divided into tenths or quadrants. Client is asked to put numbers in the appropriate places and then indicate the time as "ten minutes after eleven." Scoring is based on test used and completion of the tasks. (Manos 2004)

BATHE Technique

For a brief encounter only; keeps interview focused.
- Used when you have a very short period of time to gather information.
- Helps client identify problems and coping strategies and is supportive of client.
- Not to be used with severe problems: suicidal patients, severe abuse, and so forth (Stuart & Lieberman 1993).

■ **B**ackground - *What is going on/what brought you here?*
■ **A**ffect - *How does this make you feel?*
■ **T**rouble - *What troubles you most in your situation?*
■ **H**andling - *How are you able to handle this situation/ problem?*
■ **E**mpathy - By empathizing with client, shows an understanding of client's view of situation. Can use re-statement, paraphrasing, such as:

So this situation is making you feel sad/angry.

Ethnocultural Considerations

The following Ethnocultural Considerations table was modified from Myers 2003 with permission of the FA Davis Company. With over 400 ethnocultural groups, it is impossible to cover every group within North America. It is important, however, to become familiar with the characteristics and customs of most ethnocultural groups you will be working with and sensitive to any differences.

Ethnicity refers to a common ancestry through which individuals have evolved shared values and customs. This sense of commonality is transmitted over generations by family and reinforced by the surrounding community (Mc Goldrick 1996).

Suggested References for Further Reading Include:

Dibble S, Lipson J, and Minarik P: Culture and Nursing Care: A pocket guide. University of California, San Francisco. The Regents, 1996.

McGoldrick M, Giordano J, and Pearce JK: Ethnicity and Family Therapy, 2/e. The Guilford Press, New York 1996.

Purnell LD, and Paulanka BJ: Guide to Culturally Competent Health Care. FA Davis, Philadelphia 2004.

The International Society of Psychiatric-Mental Health Nursing position statement on *Diversity, Cultural Competence, and Access to Mental Health Care* can be accessed at: http://www.ispn-psych.org/docs/ diversityst-final.pdf

Culturally Mediated Beliefs and Practices

	Dying/Birth	Role Differences	Religion	Communication
African-American	Reluctant to donate organs	Varies by educational level/socio-economic level	Baptist/other Protestant/Muslim	*Eye Contact:* Demonstrates respect/trust *Other:* Silence may indicate distrust
Arab-American	Colostrum is believed harmful to the infant	Men make most decisions and women are responsible for daily needs	Muslim (usually Sunni)/Protestant/Greek Orthodox/other Christian	*Eye Contact:* Females may avoid eye contact with males/strangers *Other:* Supportive family members may need a break from caregiving
Asian-American	May use incense/spiritual; need extra time with deceased members	Father/eldest son primary decision maker	Primarily Buddhism and Catholicism	*Eye Contact:* Direct eye contact may be viewed as disrespectful *Other:* Use interpreters whenever possible
Native Americans	Full family involvement throughout life cycle	Varies tribe to tribe	Traditional Native American or Christian	*Eye Contact:* Eye contact sustained *Other:* American Indian may be term preferred by older adults

Culturally Mediated Beliefs and Practices

	Dying/Birth	Role Differences	Religion	Communication
Mexican-Americans	Family support during labor; very expressive during bereavement	Equal decision making with all family members	Roman Catholic primarily	*Eye Contact:* Eye contact may be avoided with authority figures *Other:* Silence may indicate disagreement with proposed plan of care
Russian-Americans	Father may not attend birth; usually closest family female does	Men and women share decision making	Eastern Orthodox and Judaism; remember recent oppression	*Eye Contact:* Direct eye contact acceptable/ nodding means approval *Other:* Use interpreters whenever possible

Adapted from Myers 2003, with permission

Perception of Mental Health Services - Ethnocultural Differences

African-Americans

■ Often distrustful of therapy and mental health services. May seek therapy because of child-focused concerns.

■ Seek help and support through "the church," which provides a sense of belonging and community (social activities/choir).

■ Understanding of therapy and mental health services. Therapy is for "crazy people" (McGoldrick 1996).

Mexican-Americans

■ Understanding the migration of the family is important, including who has been left behind. The church in the barrio often provides community support.

■ Curanderos (folk healers) may be consulted for problems such as: mal de ojo (evil eye) and susto (fright) (McGoldrick 1996).

Puerto Ricans

■ Nominally Catholic, most value the spirit and soul. Many believe in spirits that protect or harm and the value of incense and candles to ward off the "evil eye."

■ Often underutilize mental health services, and therapist needs to understand that expectations about outcome may differ (McGoldrick 1996).

Asian-American

■ Many Asian-American families are transitioning from the extended family to the nuclear unit and struggling to hold on to old ways while developing new skills.

■ Six predictors of mental health problems are: 1) employment/ financial status, 2) gender (women more vulnerable) 3) old age, 4) social isolation, 5) recent immigration, and 6) refugee premigration experiences and postmigration adjustment (McGoldrick 1996).

Above are just a few examples of many ethnocultural groups and the differences in the understanding and perception of mental health/therapy. Please refer to suggested references (p. 49) for additional and more comprehensive information.

Ethnocultural Assessment Tool

Client's name	Ethnic origin
City/State	Birth date
Significant other	Relationship
Primary language spoken	Second language
Interpreter required?	Available?
Highest level of education	Occupation

Presenting problem/
  chief complaint:

Has problem occurred before? If so how was it handled?

Client's usual manner of coping with stress?

Who is (are) client's main support system?

Family living arrangements (describe):

Major decision maker in family:

Client's/family members' roles in the family:

Religious beliefs and practices:

Are there religious restrictions or requirements?

Who takes responsibility for health in family?

Any special health concerns or beliefs?

Who does family usually approach for medical assistance?

Usual emotional/behavioral response to:

Anger _____

Anxiety _____

Pain _____

Fear _____

Loss/change/failure _____

What are sensitive topics client is unwilling to discuss because of ethnocultural taboos?

Client's feelings about touch and touching?

Client's feelings regarding eye contact?

Client's orientation to time (past/present/future)?

Illnesses/diseases common to client's ethnicity?

Client's favorite foods:

Foods that client requests or refuses because of ethnocultural reasons:

Client's perception of the problem and expectations of care and outcome:

Other:

Documentation

Problem-Oriented Record (POR)

POR	Data	Nursing Process
S (Subjective)	Client's verbal reports (e.g., "I feel nervous")	Assessment
O (Objective)	Observation (e.g., client is pacing)	Assessment
A (Assessment)	Evaluation/interpretation of S and O	Diagnosis/outcome identification
P (Plan)	Actions to resolve problem	Planning
I (Intervention)	Descriptions of actions completed	Implementation
E (Evaluation)	Reassessment to determine results and necessity of new plan of action	Evaluation

Focus Charting (DAR)

Charting	Data	Nursing Process
D (Data)	Describes observations about client/supports the stated focus	Assessment
Focus	Current client concern/ behavior/ significant change in client status	Diagnosis/outcome identification
A (Action)	Immediate/future actions	Plan and implementation
R (Response)	Client's response to care or therapy	Evaluation

Charting	Data	Nursing Process
PIE Method (APIE)		
A (Assessment)	Subjective and objective data collected at each shift	Assessment
P (Problem)	Problems being addressed from written problem list and identified outcomes	Diagnosis/outcome identification
I (Intervention)	Actions performed directed at problem resolution	Plan and implementation
E (Evaluation)	Response appraisal to determine intervention effectiveness	Evaluation

POR, DAR, and APIE were modified from Townsend 2005, with permission

CLINICAL PEARL: It is important to systematically assess and evaluate all clients and to develop a plan of action, reevaluating all assessments, plans, treatments, and outcomes. It is equally important to document all assessments, plans, treatments, and outcomes. You may "know" you provided competent treatment, but without documentation there is no record from a legal perspective. Do not ever become complacent about documentation.

Example of APIE Charting

DATE/TIME	PROBLEM:	PROGRESS NOTE:
6-22-04 1000	Social Isolation	A: States he does not want to sit with or talk to others; they "frighten him." Stays in room; no social involvement. P: Social isolation due to inability to trust. I: Spent time alone with client to initiate trust; accompanied client to group activities; praised participation. E: Cooperative although still uncomfortable in presence of group; accepted positive feedback.

Example modified from Townsend 2005, with permission.

Psychiatric Disorders

Delirium, Dementia, and Amnestic Disorders

These disorders are characterized by clinically significant cognitive deficits and notable changes from previous levels of functioning. The changes may be due to a medical condition or substance abuse or both. (APA 2000)

■ **Dementia** – Characterized *by intellectual decline and usually progressive deficits* not only in memory but also in language, perception, learning, and other areas. *Dementia of the Alzheimer's type (AD) is the most common dementia*, followed by vascular dementia (*ischemic vascular dementia*). Other causes: Infections: HIV, encephalitis, Creutzfeldt-Jackob disease; drugs and alcohol (Wernicke-Korsakoff's syndrome [thiamine deficiency]); inherited such as Parkinson's disease and Huntington's disease. Some dementias (AD) are essentially irreversible and others potentially reversible (drug toxicities, folate deficiency).

■ **Delirium** – An organic brain syndrome resulting in a *disturbance in consciousness and cognition* that happens within a short period of time with a variable course.

■ **Amnestic Disorder** – Disturbance in memory and impaired ability to learn new information or recall previously learned information.

■ **Pseudodementia** – Cognitive difficulty that is actually caused by depression, but may be mistaken for dementia. Need to consider and rule out in the elderly who may appear to have dementia when actually suffering from depression, which is a treatable disease. Could be depressed with cognitive deficits as well.

CLINICAL PEARL – AD is a progressive and irreversible dementia with a gradually declining course, whereas ischemic vascular dementia (mini-strokes and transient ischemic attacks) often presents in a stepwise fashion with an acute decline in cognitive function. It is important to distinguish between dementia and delirium because delirium can be life threatening and should be viewed as an emergency. Delirium can be differentiated from dementia by its *rapid onset, fluctuating in and out of a confusional state, and difficulty in attending to surroundings.* Delirium is usually caused by a physical condition, such as infection, and so the underlying cause needs to be treated. Keep in mind that a person with dementia may also become delirious.

Dementia of Alzheimer's Type (AD)

Signs & Symptoms	Causes	Rule Outs	Labs/Tests/Exams	Interventions
• Memory impairment • Inability to learn new material • Language deterioration (naming objects) • Inability to execute typical tasks (cook/dress self) • Executive functioning disturbances (planning/abstract thinking/new tasks) • Paranoia • Progressive from mild forgetfulness to middle and late dementia (requiring total ADL care/bedridden) • Course: 18 mo – 27 y [avg. 10–12 y]	• Idiopathic • Many theories (viral/ trauma) • Pathology shows neuritic plaques and neurofibrillary tangles; also amyloid protein • Familial AD (presenilin 1 gene) • Apolipoprotein E genotype (Kukull 2002)	• Ischemic vascular dementia • Dementia with Lewy bodies • Alcoholic dementia (Wernicke-Korsakoff [thiamine deficiency]; pellagra [niacin deficiency]; hepatic encephalitis) • Delirium • Depression • Medical disorder (HIV, syphilis) • Other substance abuse • Psychosis	• Mental status exam • Folstein Mini-Mental State Exam • Neuropsychological testing (Boston naming; Wisconsin card sorting test) • Beck Depression Inventory (R/O depression) • Geriatric Depression Scale (R/O depression) • CBC, blood chemistry (renal, metabolic/ hepatic), sed rate, T4/TSH, B_{12}-folate, UA, FTA-Abs, CT scan/ MRI; HIV titer	• Early diagnosis • Symptom treatment (aggression/ agitation) • Behavioral management • Communication techniques • Environmental safety checks • Antipsychotics • Antidepressants • Sedatives • Antianxiety agents • Nutritional supplements • Anti-Alzheimer's agents (e.g., donepezil [Aricept]; memantine [Namenda]

Dementia with Lewy Bodies

Clients with dementia with Lewy bodies usually present with visual hallucinations, and, unlike AD, the course is usually a rapid one.

ALERT: Important to differentiate AD from dementia with Lewy bodies. Clients with Lewy bodies dementia are very sensitive to antipsychotics and, because of their psychosis (visual hallucinations), are often treated with an antipsychotic. Such treatment often results in EPS. Selegiline may slow disease progression (Goroll 1995).

Medications to Treat Dementia of the Alzheimer's Type

- Medications used to treat mild to moderate AD include: tacrine [Cognex], donepezil [Aricept], and galantamine [Reminyl].
- A relatively new drug, memantine (Namenda), which is an NMDA receptor antagonist, is the first drug approved for moderate to severe AD.

Client/Family Education: Dementia

- Educate family on how to **communicate with loved ones** with dementia, especially if paranoid. Family members should not argue with someone who is agitated or paranoid.
  - Focus on positive behaviors, avoiding negative behaviors that do not pose a safety concern.
  - Avoid arguments **by talking about how the dementia client is feeling, rather than arguing the validity of a statement.** For instance, if the client says that people are coming into the house and stealing, family members can be taught to discuss *the feelings around the statement rather than the reality of it* ("That must be hard for you and we will do all we can to keep you safe").
  - Dementia clients who believe someone is stealing from them (a fixed belief) will experience even greater agitation and isolation if family members argue the point rather than recognize the feelings (fear).

- Educate family about environmental safety, as dementia clients may forget that they have turned on a stove or may have problems with balance. Throw rugs may need to be removed and stove disconnected, with family members providing meals.
- Family members need to understand that this is a **long-term management issue requiring the support of multiple health professionals and family and friends.** Management may require medication (control of hostility or for hallucinations/delusions). Remember medications need to be started at low doses and titrated slowly.
- The need for caregiver education and support cannot be underestimated. The education of the caregiver, especially if a family member, is important to help that person not overreact to sometimes difficult and threatening behaviors.
- Keep in mind that a spouse or family caregiver is also dealing with his/her own feelings of loss, helplessness, and memories of the person that once was and no longer exists.
- Teach the family caregiver how to manage difficult behaviors and situations in a calm manner, which will help both the family member and the client.
- **Caregiver stress.** Remember the caregiver also needs a break from the day-to-day stress of caring for someone with dementia. This could involve adult day care or respite provided by other family members and friends. (Chenitz et al. 1991)

Substance-Related Disorders

- Substances include prescribed medications, alcohol, over-the-counter medications, caffeine, nicotine, steroids, illegal drugs, and others; serve as central nervous system (CNS) stimulants, CNS depressants, and pain relievers; and may alter both mood and behaviors.
- Many substances are accepted by society when used in moderation (alcohol, caffeine), and others are effective in chronic pain management (opioids) but can be abused in some instances and illegal when sold on the street.
- Substance use becomes a problem when there is recurrent and persistent use despite social, work, and/or legal consequences and despite potential danger to self or others.

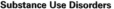

Substance Use Disorders

Substance Dependence

- Repeated use of drug despite substance-related cognitive, behavioral, and physiological problems.
- Tolerance, withdrawal, and compulsive drug-taking may result. There is a craving for the substance.
- Substance dependence does not apply to caffeine.

Substance Abuse

- Recurrent and persistent maladaptive pattern of substance use with *significant* adverse consequences occurring repeatedly or persistently during the same 12-month period.
- Repeated work absences, DUIs, spousal arguments, fights. (APA 2000)

Substance-Induced Disorders

Substance Intoxication

- Recent overuse of a substance, such as an acute alcohol intoxication, that results in a reversible, substance-specific syndrome.
- Important behavioral and psychological changes (alcohol: slurring of speech, poor coordination, impaired memory, stupor or coma).
- Can happen with one-time use of substance.

Substance Withdrawal

- Symptoms differ and are specific to each substance (cocaine, alcohol).
- Symptoms develop when a substance is discontinued after frequent substance use (anxiety, irritability, restlessness, insomnia, fatigue). (APA 2000)

Addiction, Withdrawal, & Tolerance

- *Addiction* – The repeated, compulsive use of a substance that *continues in spite of negative consequences* (physical, social, legal, etc.).
- *Physical Withdrawal/Withdrawal Syndrome* – Physiological response to the abrupt cessation or drastic reduction in a substance used (usually) for a prolonged period. The symptoms of withdrawal are specific to the substance used.
- *Tolerance* – Increased amounts of a substance over time are needed to achieve the same effect as obtained previously with smaller doses/amounts.

See Assessment Tab for CAGE Screening Questionnaire, Short Michigan Alcohol Screening Test, and Substance History and Assessment.

Substance Dependence

Signs & Symptoms	Causes	Rule Outs	Labs/Tests/Exams	Interventions
• Maladaptive coping mechanism • Clinically significant impairment/distress, same 12-mo period • Tolerance develops: increasingly larger amounts needed for same effect • Intense cravings and compulsive use; unsuccessful efforts to cut down • Inordinate time spent obtaining substance (protecting supply) • Important activities given up • Continue despite physical/psychological problems	• Genetics (hereditary, esp. alcohol) • Biochemical • Psychosocial • Ethnocultural • Need to approach as biopsychosocial disorder • Response to substances can be very individualistic	• Consider co-morbidities: Mood disorders, such as bipolar/depression: ECA study: (Reiger et al, 1990) 60.7% diagnosed with bipolar I had lifetime diagnosis of substance use disorders • Untreated chronic pain • Undiagnosed depression in elderly (isolation a problem)	• CAGE question-naire • SMAST, others • Toxicology screens (emergencies) • Beck Depression Inventory (R/O depression) • GDS • Labs: LFTs – γ-glutamyl-transferase (GGT) and mean corpuscular volume (MCV); %CDT (carbohydrate-deficient trans-ferrin) (Anton 2001)	• Early identification and education • Confidential and nonjudgmental approach • Evaluate for co-morbidities and treat other disorders • Evaluate own attitudes about substance use/dependence • Psychotherapy • Behavior therapy • 12-step programs • Medications: mood stabilizers, antidepressants, naltrexone • Detoxification • Hospitalization

Client/Family Education: Substance-Related Disorders

■ Keep in mind that most clients underestimate their substance use (especially alcohol consumption) and that denial is the usual defense mechanism.

■ When substance dependence/abuse is suspected, it is important to approach the client in a supportive and nonjudgmental manner. Focus on the consequences of continued substance use and abuse (physically/emotionally/family/employment) and discuss the need for complete abstinence.
For a client to stop any substance abuse, he/she must first recognize and accept that there is a problem. It requires a desire and commitment on the part of the client to stop the substance use. Even with a desire, there can be relapses.

■ If a substance user/abuser will not seek help, then family members should be encouraged to seek help through organizations such as AlAnon (families of alcoholics) or NarAnon (families of narcotic addicts). AlaTeen is for adolescent children of alcoholics, and Adult Children of Alcoholics (ACOA) is for adults who grew up with alcoholic parents.

■ For substance abusers, there are Alcoholics Anonymous, Narcotics Anonymous, Overeaters Anonymous, Smokers Anonymous, Women for Sobriety, etc. There is usually a support group available to deal with the unique issues of each addiction.

■ In some instances, medication may be required to manage the withdrawal phase (physical dependence) of a substance. Benzodiazepines may be needed, including inpatient detoxification (Goroll 1995). Cocaine abusers may be helped with desipramine, fluoxetine, or amantadine (Antai-Otong 2003).

■ Naltrexone, an opioid antagonist, reduces cravings by blocking opioid receptors in the brain and is used in heroin addiction and alcohol addiction (reduces cravings and number of drinking days) (Tai 2004; Maxman & Ward 1995).

■ Substance-related disorders can be difficult to treat, but there are many trained substance abuse and addiction specialists as well as support groups and medications available to those with a desire to abstain. Educate clients and families about the possibility of co-morbidities (bipolar disease) and the need to treat these disorders as well.

Schizophrenia and Other Psychotic Disorders

In 1908, **Eugen Bleuler**, a Swiss psychiatrist, introduced the term **schizophrenia**, which replaced the term dementia praecox, used by **Emil Kraepelin** (1896). Kraepelin viewed this disorder as a deteriorating organic disease; Bleuler viewed it as a serious disruption of the mind, a "splitting of the mind." In 1948, **From-Reichman** coined the term **schizophrenogenic mother**, described as cold and domineering, although appearing self-sacrificing. **Bateson** (1973, 1979) introduced the **double bind**, wherein the child *could never win* and was always wrong (invalidation disguised as acceptance; illusion of choice; paradoxical communication).

- **Schizophrenia is a complex disorder**, and it is now accepted that schizophrenia is the result of neurobiological factors rather than due to some early psychological trauma.
  - The **lifetime prevalence rate** (US/worldwide) is about 1%.
  - Onset in the late teens to early 20s, equally affecting men and women.
  - Devastating disease for both the client and the family.
  - Schizophrenia affects thoughts and emotions to the point that social and occupational functioning is impaired (Kessler 1994; Bromet 1995).
  - About 9% to 13% of schizophrenics commit suicide (Meltzer 2003).

- **Early diagnosis and treatment are critical** to slowing the deterioration and decline that will result without treatment.
  - Earlier typical antipsychotics effective against most of the positive symptoms; less effective against negative symptoms.
  - Atypical antipsychotics work on both negative and positive symptoms.
  - Family/community support is key factor in improvement.

- **Subtypes of schizophrenia** include paranoid, disorganized, catatonic, undifferentiated, and residual types.

- **National Association for the Mentally Ill** (www.nami.org) is an important national organization that has done much to educate society and communities about mental illness and to advocate for the seriously mentally ill.

- **Other psychotic disorders** include schizophreniform disorder, schizoaffective disorder, delusional disorder, brief psychotic disorder, shared psychotic disorder (folie à deux), psychotic disorder due to a medical condition, substance induced, and NOS.

Schizophrenia

Signs & Symptoms	Causes	Rule Outs	Labs/Tests/Exams	Interventions
• At least for 1 month, 2 or more from the following: ◆ Delusions ◆ Hallucinations ◆ Disorganized speech ◆ Disorganized behavior ◆ Negative symptoms (alogia, affective flattening, avolition) • Functional disturbances at school, work, self care, personal relations • Disturbance continues for 6 mo	• Dopamine hypothesis (excess) • Brain abnormalities (3rd ventricle sometimes larger) • Frontal lobe – decreased glucose use/smaller frontal lobe • Genetic – familial; monozygotic twin (47% risk vs 12% dizygotic) • Virus • No specific cause	• Schizophreniform disorder • Schizoaffective • Mood disorder with psychotic symptoms • Medical • Substance/substance abuse with psychotic episode • Delusional disorder • Note: With schizophrenia, the condition persists for at least 6 mo and is chronic and deteriorating	• Psychiatric evaluation and mental status exam • No test can diagnose schizophrenia • Positive and Negative Syndrome Scale (PANSS) • Abnormal Involuntary Movement Scale (AIMS) • Need to rule out other possible medical/substance use disorders: LFTs, toxicology screens, CBC, TFT, CT scan, etc.	• Antipsychotic – usually atypicals for new onset: risperidone, olanzapine, aripiprazole, etc. • Acute psychotic episode may need high potency (haloperidol) • Hospitalization until positive symptoms under control • Patient/family education • NAMI for patient/family education, as patient advocate

Positive and Negative Symptoms of Schizophrenia

■ Positive Symptoms

Positive symptoms are excesses in behavior (excessive function/distortions)

- Delusions
- Hallucinations (auditory/visual)
- Hostility
- Disorganized thinking/behaviors

■ Negative Symptoms

Negative symptoms are deficits in behavior (reduced function; self care deficits)

- Alogia
- Affective blunting
- Anhedonia
- Asociality
- Avolition
- Apathy

Four A's of Schizophrenia

■ Eugen Bleuler in 1911 proposed four basic diagnostic areas for characterizing schizophrenia. These became the 4 A's:

A: Inappropriate **Affect**
A: Loosening of **Associations**
A: **Autistic** Thoughts
A: **Ambivalence**

■ These four A's provide a memory tool for recalling how schizophrenia affects thinking, mood (flat), thought processes, and decision-making ability. (Shader 1994)

CLINICAL PEARL – When auditory hallucinations first begin, they usually sound soft and far away and eventually become louder. When the sounds become soft and distant again, the auditory hallucinations are usually abating. The majority of hallucinations in North America are auditory (versus visual) and it is unlikely that a client will experience both auditory and visual hallucinations at the same time.

Thought Disorders – Content of Thought (Definitions)

Common Delusions

Delusion of Grandeur – Exaggerated/unrealistic sense of importance, power, identity. *Thinks he/she is the President or Jesus Christ.*

Delusion of Persecution –Others are out to harm or persecute in some way. *May believe their food is being poisoned or they are being watched.*

Delusion of Reference – Everything in the environment is somehow related to the person. *A television news broadcast has a special message for this person solely.*

Somatic Delusion – An unrealistic belief about the body, such as *the brain is rotting away.*

Control Delusion – Someone or something is controlling the person. *Radio towers are transmitting thoughts and telling person what to do.*

Thought Disorders – Form of Thought (Definitions)

Circumstantiality – Excessive and irrelevant detail in descriptions with the person eventually making his/her point. *We went to a new restaurant. The waiter wore several earrings and seemed to walk with a limp...yes, we loved the restaurant.*

Concrete Thinking – Unable to abstract and speaks in concrete, literal terms. *For instance, a rolling stone gathers no moss would be interpreted literally.*

Clang Association – Association of words by sound rather than meaning. *She cried till she died but could not hide from the ride.*

Loose Association – A loose connection between thoughts that are often unrelated. *The bed was unmade. She went down the hill and rolled over to her good side. And the flowers were planted there.*

Tangentiality – Digressions in conversation from topic to topic and the person never makes his/her point. *Went to see Joe the other day. By the way, bought a new car. Mary hasn't been around lately.*

Neologism – Creation of a new word meaningful only to that person. *The hiphopmobilly is on its way.*

Word Salad – Combination of words that have no meaning or connection. *Inside outside blue market calling.*

Client/Family Education: Schizophrenia

- Both client and family education are critical to improve chances of relapse prevention, to slow or prevent regression as well as associated long-term disability.
- Refer client/family to the National Association for the Mentally III (NAMI) (www.nami.org) (1-800-950-NAMI [6264]) and National Schizophrenia Foundation (www.NSFoundation.org) (800-482-9534).
- Client and family need to be educated about the importance of taking antipsychotic medication to prevent relapse. Client will likely need medication indefinitely to prevent relapse and possible worsening of condition.
- Client needs both medication and family/community support. Studies have shown that clients taking medication can still relapse if living with high expressed emotion family members (spouse/parent). These family members are critical, intense, hostile, and overly involved versus low expressed emotion family members (Davies 1994).
- Once stabilized on medication, clients often stop taking their medication because they feel they no longer need their medica- tion (denying the illness or believing they have recovered). It is important to stress the need for medication indefinitely and that maintenance medication is needed to prevent relapse.
- Clients also stop medication because of untoward side effects. Engage the client in a discussion about medications, so that he/she has some control about medication options. The newer atypicals have a better side effect profile, but it is important to listen to the client's concerns (weight gain/EPS) as adjustments are possible or a switch to another medication. Educate client/family that periodic lab tests will be needed.
- Some antipsychotics result in weight gain, so advise client to monitor food intake and provide dietary education as needed. Weighing weekly at first may anticipate a problem early on or for institution of a diet and exercise. ALERT: For those on antipsychotic therapy, there is also now a concern with treatment-emergent diabetes, especially for those with risk factors for diabetes, such as family history, obesity, and glucose intolerance (Buse et al. 2002).

■ Early diagnosis, early treatment, and ongoing antipsychotic maintenance therapy with family support are critical factors in slowing the progression of this disease and in keeping those with schizophrenia functional and useful members of society.

Mood Disorders

A **mood disorder** is related to a person's emotional tone or affective state and can have an effect on behavior and can influence a person's personality and world view.

■ Extremes of mood (mania or depression) can have devastating consequences on client, family, and society alike.
■ These consequences include financial, legal, marital, relationship, employment, and spiritual losses as well as despair that results in potential suicide and death.
■ Correct diagnosis is needed, and effective treatments are available.

The **mood disorders** are divided into *depressive disorders* and *bipolar disorders*.

■ The **depressive disorders** include major depressive disorder, dysthymic disorder, and depressive disorder NOS.
■ The **bipolar disorders** include bipolar I disorder, bipolar II disorder, cyclothymic disorder, and bipolar disorder NOS.

Depressive Disorders

■ **Major depressive disorder** (unipolar depression) requires at least 2 weeks of depression/loss of interest and 4 additional depressive symptoms, with one or more major depressive episodes.
■ **Dysthymic disorder** is an ongoing low-grade depression of at least 2 years' duration for more days than not and does not meet the criteria for major depression.
■ **Depression NOS** does not meet the criteria for major depression and other disorders. (APA 2000)

Bipolar Disorders

- **Bipolar I disorder** includes one or more manic or mixed episodes, usually with a major depressive episode.
- **Bipolar II disorder** includes one or two major depressive episodes and at least one hypomanic (less than full mania) episode.
- **Cyclothymic disorder** includes at least 2 years of hypomanic periods that do not meet the criteria for the other disorders.
- **Bipolar NOS** does not meet any of the other bipolar criteria.
- **Others:** Mood disorders due to a general medical condition, substance-induced mood disorders, and mood disorder NOS. (APA 2000).

SIGECAPS – Mnemonic for Depression

Following is a mnemonic for easy recall and review of the DSM-IV criteria for **major depression or dysthymia**:

Sleep (increase/decrease)
Interest (diminished)
Guilt/low self esteem
Energy (poor/low)
Concentration (poor)
Appetite (increase/decrease)
Psychomotor (agitation/retardation)
Suicidal ideation

A depressed mood for 2 or more weeks, plus 4 SIGECAPS = major depressive disorder

A depressed mood, plus 3 SIGECAPS for 2 years, most days = dysthymia (Brigham and Women's Hospital 2001)

CLINICAL PEARL – Important to determine that a depressive episode is a unipolar depression versus a bipolar disorder with a *depressive episode*. A first depressive episode 1 or II may begin with major depression. The presentation is a "clinical snapshot in time" rather than the complete picture. Further evaluation and monitoring is needed. Bipolar clients are often misdiagnosed for years.

- One study (Ghaemi et al. 2003) showed 37% of patients were misdiag-nosed (depression versus bipolar), resulting in new or worsening rapid cycling (mania) in 23%, because antidepressants were prescribed (Keck 2003).
- Although the tricyclic antidepressants (TCAs) are more likely to trigger a manic episode, the SSRIs have also been implicated.

ALERT: If a client who is recently prescribed antidepressants begins showing manic symptoms, consider that this client may be bipolar.

Major Depressive Episode				
Signs & Symptoms	Causes	Rule Outs	Labs/Tests/Exams	Interventions
• Depressed mood or loss of interest for at least 2 weeks & 5 or more of: ♦ Significant weight loss/gain ♦ Insomnia or hypersomnia ♦ Psychomotor agitation or retardation ♦ Fatigue ♦ Worthless feelings or inappropriate guilt ♦ Problem concentrating ♦ Recurrent thoughts of death	• Familial predisposition • Deficiency of norepinephrine • Hypothalamic dysfunction; serotonin and norepinephrine • Thyroid/adrenal dysfunction: hypothyroidism • Neoplasms • CNS (stroke) • Vitamin deficiencies (folic acid) • Psychosocial factors • Unknown	• Bipolar I or II disorder • Schizoaffective • Grief (major loss) (female is 3:1 male, 3:1) (acute distress → 3 mo) • Postpartum depression • Medication (reserpine, prednisone) • Pseudodementia (older adult) • Substance abuse disorder (cocaine)	• Psychiatric evaluation and mental status exam • Beck Depression Inventory (BDI); Zung Self-Rating Scale; Geriatric Depression Scale • MMSE • Physical exam • Rule out other possible medical/substance use disorders: LFTs, toxicology screens, CBC, TFT, CT scan, etc.	• Antidepressants: usually SSRIs (fluoxetine, sertraline); SNRIs (venlafaxine [includes norepinephrine]) TCAs: side effects include sedation, dry mouth, blurred vision; helpful for sleep (trazodone [priapism]); TCAs not good for elderly (falls) • Others: Bupropion • MAOIs • Cognitive-behavioral therapy • Psychotherapy • ECT

Manic Episode

Signs & Symptoms	Causes	Rule Outs	Labs/Tests/Exams	Interventions
• Persistent elevated, irritable mood ≥ 1 wk, plus 3 or more (irritable, 4 or more): ◆ ↑self esteem ◆ ↓sleep ◆ ↑talk/pressured speech ◆ racing thoughts/ flight of ideas ◆ distractibility ◆ extreme goal-directed activity ◆ excessive buying/sex/business investments (painful consequences)	• Genetic: famil-ial predisposi-tion (female to male, 1.2:1) • Bipolar onset 18 – 20 yr • Catechola-mines: norep-inephrine, dopamine • Many hypotheses: serotonin, acetylcholine; neuroanato-mical (front-otemporal lesions); • Complex disorder	• Hypomanic episode (bipolar II) • Mixed episode (major depressive and manic episode ≥1 wk) • Cyclothymia • Substance induced (cocaine) • Dual diagnosis • ADHD • Brain lesion • General medical condition	• Psychiatric evaluation and mental status exam • Young Mania Rating Scale (YMRS) (Bipolar I) • Need to rule out other possible medical/sub-stance use/induced disorders: LFTs, toxicology screens, CBC, TFT, CT scan, etc.	• Mood stabi-lizers: lithium (standard); anticonvul-sants (carba-mazepine, valproic acid, lamotrigine) • Combined treatments: Lithium & anticonvul-sant • Lithium: + for mania/not for mixed • Therapy & medication compliance

Postpartum Major Depressive Episode

Signs & Symptoms	Causes	Rule Outs	Labs/Tests/Exams	Interventions
• Symptoms similar to major depressive episode • Acute onset to slowly over 1st three postpartum (PP) months • Persistent/debilitating mood, tearfulness, insomnia, suicidal thoughts • Depressed mood, Anxiety, obsession about well being of infant • Affects functioning	• Occurs in 10 – 15% of women • Highest risk: hx of depression, previous PP depression; ends 2 weeks; depression during pregnancy • Previous PP depression with psychosis: ↑ risk of recurrence at subsequent delivery	• PP blues: (fluctuating mood; peaks 4th d post delivery; questionnaire functioning intact) • PP psychosis: 1 – 2/1000 women; ↑ risk: bipolar/ prev PP psychosis; infanticide/ suicide risk high • R/O medical cause	• Edinburgh Postnatal Depression Scale (EPDS): self rated questionnaire • Screen during PP period • Psychiatric evaluation • Physical exam • Routine lab tests: CBC, TFT (thyroid/anemia)	• Pharmacologic: SSRIs, SNRIs, TCAs (insomnia; consider weight gain, dry mouth, sedation with TCAs • CBT, individual, group psychotherapy • Anxiolytics • ECT • Psychosis: hospitalization; mood stabilizers, antipsychotics, ECT

Client/Family Education: Mood Disorders

Mood disorders can range from subthreshold to mild (dysthymic) to extreme (manic/psychotic) fluctuations in emotion and behaviors.

Family and client need educating about the specific disorder, whether major depression, bipolar I or II, postpartum depression, or unresolved grief. Without treatment, support, and education, the results can be devastating emotionally, interpersonally, legally, and financially.

- The mood disorders need to be explained in terms of their biochemical basis – "depression is an illness, not a weakness," although often recurrent, chronic illnesses.

- Families and clients need to understand that early diagnosis and treatment are essential for effective management and improved outcome.

- It may be helpful to compare to other chronic illnesses, such as diabetes and asthma, as a model and to reinforce the biological basis of the illness to reduce stigmatism. As with any chronic illness (diabetes, asthma), on-going management, including pharmacologic treatment, is required.

- Reinforce the need to adhere to the dosing schedule as prescribed and not to make any unilateral decisions, including stopping, without conferring with health professional.

- There may be exacerbations from time to time with a need to modify treatment. Help client and family identify early signs of regression, and advise to immediately contact the health professional in charge.

- Work with client and family on side effect management. If client can be part of the decision making when there are options, client will be more willing to become involved in own recovery and continue treatment.

- Address weight gain possibilities (lithium, anticonvulsants, antipsychotics); monitor weight, BMI, exercise and food plans to prevent weight gain.

Death and Dying/Grief

Stages of Death and Dying (Kübler-Ross)

1. *Denial and Isolation* – usually temporary state of being unable to accept the possibility of one's death or that of a loved one.
2. *Anger* – replacement of temporary "stage one" with the reality that death is possible/going to happen. This is the realization that the future (plans/hopes) will have an end; a realization of the finality of the self. May fight/argue with health care workers/push family/friends away.
3. *Bargaining* – seeks one last hope or possibility. Enters an agreement or pact with God for "one last time or event" to take place before death. (Let me live to see my grandchild born or my child graduate from college.)
4. *Depression* – after time, loss, pain, the person realizes the situation and course of illness will not improve. Necessary stage to reach acceptance.
5. *Acceptance* – after working/passing through the previous stages, the person finally accepts what is going to happen. This is not resignation (giving up) or denying and fighting to the very end. It is a stage that allows for peace and dignity. (Kübler-Ross 1997)

Complicated versus Uncomplicated Grief

Complicated Grief	Uncomplicated Grief
• Excessive in duration (may be delayed reaction or compounded losses [multiple losses]); usually longer than 3 – 6 mo • Disabling symptoms, morbid preoccupation with deceased/physical symptoms • Substance abuse, increased alcohol intake • Risk factors: Limbo states (missing person), ambivalent relationship, multiple losses; long-term partner (sole dependency); no social network; history of depression • Suicidal thoughts – may want to join the deceased	• Follows a major loss • Depression perceived as normal • Self esteem intact • Guilt specific to lost one (should have telephoned more) • Distress usually resolves within 12 weeks (though mourning can continue for 1 or more years) • Suicidal thoughts transient or unusual (Shader 1994)

Anxiety Disorders

- The **anxiety disorders** include a wide range of disorders from the very specific, such as phobias, to generalized anxiety disorder, which is pervasive and experienced as dread or apprehension.
- Other anxiety disorders include panic disorder, agoraphobia (avoidance of places that may result in panic), social phobia, obsessive-compulsive disorder, posttraumatic stress disorder, acute stress disorder, anxiety due to a medical disorder, substance-induced anxiety disorder, and anxiety disorder NOS.
- Some anxiety is good, motivates us to perform at our best.
- **Excessive anxiety** can be crippling and may result in the "fight or flight" reaction. The *fighter* is ever ready for some perceived aggression and may avoid upsetting situations or actually freezes with anxiety and is unable to relax, and the *escaper (flight)* freezes with anxiety and may avoid upsetting situations or actually dissociate (leave their body/fragment).
- Either extreme is not good and can result in physical and emotional exhaustion. (See Fight-or-Flight Response and Stress Adaptation Syndrome in Basics Tab.)

Four Levels of Anxiety

- *Mild Anxiety* – This is the anxiety that can positively motivate someone to perform at a high level. It helps a person to focus on the situation at hand. For instance, this kind of anxiety is often experienced by performers before entering the stage.
- *Moderate Anxiety* – Anxiety now moves up a notch with narrowing of the perceptual field. The person has trouble attending to his/her surroundings, although he/she can follow commands/direction.
- *Severe Anxiety* – Increasing anxiety brings the person to yet another level, resulting in an inability to attend to his/her surroundings, except for maybe a detail. Physical symptoms may develop, such as sweating and palpitations (pounding heart). Anxiety relief is the goal.
- *Panic Anxiety* – The level reached is now one of terror where the only concern is to escape. Communication impossible at this point. (Peplau 1963)

CLINICAL PEARL – Recognizing level of anxiety is important in determining intervention. Important to manage anxiety before it escalates. At the moderate level, firm, short, direct commands are needed: *You need to sit down, Mr. Jones.*

Generalized Anxiety Disorder (GAD)

Signs & Symptoms	Causes	Rule Outs	Labs/Tests/Exams	Interventions
• Excessive anxiety; at least 6 mo; difficult to control worry/hypervigilant	• Neurotransmitter dysregulation: NE, 5-HT, GABA	• Anxiety disorder due to a medical condition (hyperthyroidism; pheochromocytoma)	• Self-rated scales: Beck Anxiety Inventory (BAI); State Trait Anxiety Inventory	• Pharmacologic: Benzodiazepines very effective (diazepam, lorazepam); nonbenzodiazepines: buspirone
• Associated with 3 or more: ❖ Restless/on edge ❖ Easily fatigued ❖ Concentration problems ❖ Irritability ❖ Muscle tension ❖ Sleep disturbance	• Autonomic nervous system activation: locus ceruleus/NE release/limbic system	• Substance induced anxiety or caffeine-induced anxiety	• Observer-rated scale: Hamilton Anxiety Rating Scale (HAM-A)	
• Causes significant distress	• One year prevalence rate: 1%; lifetime prevalence, 5%	• Other anxiety disorders: panic disorder, OCD, etc.; DSM-IV criteria help rule out	• Psychiatric evaluation	• Beta-blockers: propranolol
• Often physical complaints: dizziness, tachycardia, tightness of chest, sweating, tremor	• Familial association		• Physical exam	• Deep muscle relaxation
	• Over half: onset in childhood		• Routine lab tests; TFTs	• CBT
				• Individual and family therapy
				• Education

Obsessive-Compulsive Disorder (OCD)

Signs & Symptoms	Causes	Rule Outs	Labs/Tests/Exams	Interventions
• *Obsessions* – recurrent, intrusive thoughts that cause anxiety OR *Compulsions* – repetitive behaviors (hand washing, checking) that reduce distress/anxiety and must be adhered to rigidly • Driven to perform compulsions • Time consuming (>1 hr/d), interfere with normal routine • Recognizes thoughts/behaviors are unreasonable	• Genetic evidence • Neurobiological basis: orbito-frontal cortex, cingulate, and caudate nucleus • Neurochemical: serotonergic and possibly dopaminergic • Association between OCD and Tourette's, and others • Lifetime prevalence of 2.5% • Women > men • Avg onset: 20 y • Childhood: 7 – 10 y	• Other anxiety disorders: phobias • Impulse control disorders • Obsessive-compulsive personality disorder • Body dysmorphic disorder • Depression • Neuro-logical disorders	• Yale-Brown Obsessive Compulsive Scale (Y-BOCS) • Psychiatric evaluation • Mental status exam • Neurologic exam	• Pharmaco-logic: SSRIs (fluoxetine: higher doses); fluvoxamine; clomipramine • Beta-blockers: propranolol • Behavior therapy: exposure and response prevention • Deep muscle relaxation • Individual & family therapy • Education

Posttraumatic Stress Disorder (PTSD)

Signs & Symptoms	Causes	Rule Outs	Labs/Tests/Exams	Interventions
• Traumatic event (self/family/witness others); threat of harm or death or actual death and helplessness	• Rape, torture, child abuse, disaster, war, etc.	• Acute stress disorder (clinician administered)	• PTSD scale (clinician administered)	• Debriefing (rescuers, etc.)
• Reexperiencing event "flash-backs" (triggers: sounds/smell)	• Physiologic/neurochemical/endocrinological alterations	• Obsessive-compulsive disorder	• Psychiatric evaluation	• Individual or group psychotherapy
• Hypervigilance/recurrent nightmares/ numbing	• Sympathetic hyperarousal	• Adjustment disorder	• Mental status exam	• CBT
• Anniversary reactions (unaware reenactment related to trauma)	• Limbic system (amygdala dysfunction)	• Depression	• Neurologic exam	• EMDR (Eye Movement Desensitization & Reprocessing) (Shapiro 1995)
• Persistent anxiety/outbursts	• "Kindling": ↑ neuronal excitability	• Panic disorder	• CAGE, SMAST	• Pharmacotherapy: Antidepressants– SSRIs, SNRIs, MAOIs, TCAs; antipsychotics; anxiolytics; mood stabilizers
• Acute (<3 mo); chronic (≥3 mo); delayed (>6 mo)	• Risk factor: previous trauma	• Psychotic disorder	• Physical exam, routine blood studies	• Family and community support/art therapy/psychodrama
	• Lifetime prevalence ~8% (US)	• Substance-induced disorder	• No laboratory test can diagnose	
		• Psychotic disorder due to a general medical condition		
		• Delirium		

Client/Family Education: Anxiety Disorders

Anxiety, the most common disorder in the US, exists along a continuum and may be in response to a specific stressor (taking a test), or it may present as a generalized "free floating" anxiety (GAD) or a panic disorder (PD) (feeling of terror). A 1-year prevalence rate for all anxieties has been said to be in the 5 – 15% range (Shader 1994).

- Most people have experienced some degree of anxiety, and so it might be helpful for family members to understand the 4 stages of anxiety and how one stage builds on the other – especially in trying to explain panic disorder.
- It is important for families to understand the importance of early diagnosis and treatment of anxiety disorders, as these are chronic illnesses and will become worse and more difficult to treat over time.
- Explain to client and family the need for ongoing management (pharmacological/education/psychotherapeutic/cognitive-behavioral therapy [CBT], *just as diabetes and asthma and heart disease must be managed.*
- Many of these disorders are frustrating to family members. It is hard to understand the repetitive handwashing or checking that can be done by someone with OCD. Family members are also affected, and the client's illness becomes a family issue as well.
- The client may also need to be educated about the needs of other family members (maybe time away from client). Family therapy may be needed to negotiate and agree on living arrangements in a way that respects the needs of the client and all family members.
- As in all chronic disorders, remissions and exacerbations will be experienced. At times reinforcement sessions (CBT) are needed, especially with CBT and exposure/response prevention for OCD.
- Remind families that patience, persistence, and a multimodal/multiteam approach to treatment are needed.
- Reinforce with families that they also need support and sometimes a respite from the situation.
- Helpful to give a family member "permission" to take a respite and express own needs/frustrations, as well as positive feelings toward client.

Sexual and Gender Identity Disorders

The Sexual and Gender Identity Disorders are divided into three main categories by the DSM-IV-TR. But in order to understand dysfunction, we first need to understand and define sexual health.

- *Sexual health* is defined as a state of physical, emotional, mental, and social well being related to sexuality; it is not merely the absence of disease or dysfunction. It requires a respectful and positive approach, free of coercion, discrimination, and violence. Sexual practices are safe and have the possibility of pleasure (WHO 1975).
- A person's *sex* refers to *biological* characteristics that define this person as a male or a female (some individuals possess both male and female biological characteristics [hermaphrodite/intersex]) (WHO 2002).
- *Gender* refers to the characteristics of men and women that are *socially constructed,* rather than biologically determined. We are taught the *behaviors* and *roles* that result in our becoming men and women, also known as *gender identity* and *gender roles.*
  - ◆ Gender roles are also culturally determined and differ from one culture to another; they are not static; they are also affected by the law and religious practice.
  - ◆ Gender also relates to power relationships (between men and women) as well as reproductive rights issues and responsibilities (APA 2000).
- *Sexual orientation* refers to the sexual preference of a person, whether male to female, female to female, male to male, or bisexual. Variations in sexual preference are considered to be sexually healthy (APA 2000).

Sexual Dysfunctions

- *Sexual dysfunction* is a disturbance in the sexual response cycle or is associated with pain during intercourse.
- *Sexual response cycle dysfunctions* include the areas of desire, excitement, orgasm, and resolution. Categories include: hypoactive sexual desire disorder, sexual aversion disorder, female sexual arousal disorder, male erectile disorder, female and male orgasmic disorders, and premature ejaculation.

■ The *pain disorders* include: dyspareunia, vaginismus, sexual function due to a medical disorder, substance-induced sexual dysfunction, and sexual dysfunction NOS.

Paraphilias

■ The *paraphilias* are sexually arousing fantasies, urges, or behaviors triggered by/focused on nonhuman objects, self or partner humiliation, nonconsenting adults, or children that are recurrent for a period of at least 6 months.

■ There are episodic paraphilias that operate only during times of stress.

■ *Paraphilias* include *pedophilia* (sexual activity with a child ≤ 13 y); *frotteurism* (touching/rubbing nonconsenting person); *fetishism* (nonhuman object used for/needed for arousal); *exhibitionism* (genital exposure to a stranger); *voyeurism* (observing unsuspecting persons naked or in sexual activity); *sexual masochism* (humiliation/suffering) and *sadism* (excitement from inflicting suffering/humiliation); and others. (APA 2000)

Gender Identity Disorder

■ **Gender Identity Disorder** requires a *cross-gender identification* and a belief and insistence that "one is the other sex." The desire is persistent, and the preference is for cross-sex roles. Prefer the stereotypical roles and games/pastimes/clothing of other sex.

■ There exists an extreme and persistent discomfort with the biological sex at birth and the sense of oneself as not belonging to the gender role of the biological sex.

■ Boys will have an aversion to own penis and testicles, and girls resent growing breasts or female clothing.

■ This is not a physical intersex condition, and there is definite distress over the biological sex that affects important areas of functioning. (APA 2000)

Because sexuality and its dysfunctions involve cultural considerations and attitudes, moral and ethical concerns, religious beliefs, as well as legal considerations, it is important to evaluate your own beliefs, values, possible prejudices, and comfort level in dealing with sexual disorders.

Hypoactive Sexual Desire Disorder

Signs & Symptoms	Causes	Rule Outs	Labs/Tests/Exams	Interventions
• Deficiency or absence of sexual fantasies or desires; persistent/recurrent • Marked distress/interpersonal difficulties • Not substance-induced or due to a general medical condition • Does not usually initiate sex and reluctantly engages in sex with partner • Relationship/marital difficulties • Lifelong/acquired/situational	• Psychological: partner incompatibility, anger, sexual identity issues, sexual preference issues, negative parental views (as a child)	• Sexual aversion disorder (intense fear/disgust over sex vs disinterest) • Extremes in sexual appetite (sexual addict as a partner) • Major depression • Medical condition • Substance abuse • Medication • Sexual abuse • Other	• Complete physical exam, including medical history • Psychiatric evaluation • Mental status exam • Sexual history • Routine lab work • BDI • Zung • CAGE • SMAST • TFT	• Refer to sex therapist • Relationship therapy • CBT • Assuming no physical/medication/substance use disorder, deal with relationship issues and assure sexual compatibility and sexual orientation

Client/Family Education: Sexual Dysfunctions/Paraphilias/
Gender Identity Disorders

Sexual Dysfunctions

■ Clients and their partners need to understand where in the sexual response cycle the problem exists (arousal/orgasm).

■ If the problem is one of desire or aversion, this needs to be explored further to determine the causes: couple discord, gender identity or sexual orientation issues, negative views of sexual activity, previous sexual abuse, body image or self-esteem issues!

■ The same holds true for other sexual dysfunctions (orgasmic problems/erectile dysfunction) in that issues around substance use/abuse, previous sexual experiences, possible psychological, physical, and other stressors as factors, including medical conditions and prescribed medications, need to be explored.

■ Referral to a sex therapist may be needed to find ways to reconnect intimately. Sometimes partner education is needed on how to satisfy the other partner (mutual satisfaction).

Paraphilias and Gender Identity Disorders

The **Paraphilias** and **Gender Identity Disorders** require help from those professionals especially trained in dealing with these disorders. Clients and families need to receive support and education from these professionals.

Eating Disorders

■ Eating disorders are influenced by many factors, including family rituals and values around food and eating, ethnic and cultural influences, societal influences, and individual biology.

■ American society currently stresses physical beauty and fitness and favors the thin and slim female as the ideal.

■ There has been a dramatic increase in the number of obese people in the United States – at an alarming rate among children.

■ With society's emphasis on fast and convenient foods, high in calories, a reduction in exercise (computers/TV), and the ongoing value of "thin as beautiful," eating disorders remain a concern.

Anorexia Nervosa/Bulimia Nervosa

- Two specific eating disorders are **anorexia nervosa (AN)** and **bulimia nervosa (BN)**. (*For BN see Table that follows.*) Both use/manipulate eating behaviors in an effort to control weight. Each has its dangers and consequences if maintained over time.
- *Anorexia Nervosa* – The anorexia nervosa client is terrified of gaining weight and does not maintain a minimally acceptable body weight.
  - ◆ There is a definite disturbance in the perception of the size or shape of the body.
  - ◆ AN is more common in the industrialized societies and can begin as early as age 13.
  - ◆ Body weight in the anorexic client is less than 85% of what would be expected for that age and height.
  - ◆ Even though underweight, client still fears becoming overweight.
  - ◆ Self-esteem and self-evaluation based on weight and body shape.
  - ◆ Amenorrhea develops, as defined by absence of three consecutive menstrual cycles (see bulimia nervosa). (APA 2000)

Client/Family Education: Eating Disorders

- Client and family need to understand the serious nature of both disorders; mortality rate for AN is 2 – 8% (30 – 40% recover; 25 – 30% improve; 15 – 20% do not improve). About 50% of BN recover with treatment. (Rakel 2000)
- *Team approach important* – client and family need to be involved with the team, which should or may include a nutritionist, psychiatrist, therapist, physician, psychiatric nurse, nurse, eating disorder specialist, and others.
- Teach client coping strategies, allow for expression of feelings, teach relaxation techniques, and help with ways (other than food) to feel in control.
- Family therapy important to work out parent-child issues, especially around control (should have experience with eating disorders).
- Focus on the fact that clients do recover and improve, and encourage patience when there is a behavioral setback.

Bulimia Nervosa (BN)

Signs & Symptoms	Causes	Rule Outs	Labs/Tests/Exams	Interventions
• Recurrent binge eating of large amount of food over short time period • Lack of control and cannot stop • Self-induced vomiting, laxatives, (purging) fasting, exercise(nonpurging) to compensate • At least 2 X/w for 3 mo • Normal weight, some underweight/overweight • Tooth enamel erosion/finger or pharynx bruising • F & E disturbances	• Genetic predisposition • Hypothalamic dysfunction implication • Family hx of mood disorders and obesity • Issues of power and control • Societal emphasis on thin • Affects 1 – 3% women • Develops late adolescence through adulthood	• Anorexia nervosa, binge-eating, purging type • MDD with atypical features • Borderline PD • General medical conditions: Kleine-Levin syndrome • Endocrine disorders	• Complete physical exam • Psychiatric evaluation • Mental status exam • Routine lab work, including TFT, CBC, electrolytes, UA • ECG • CAGE • SMAST	• Individual, group, marital, family therapy • Behavior modification • Nutritional support • Medical support • Client-family education

Personality Disorders

- When a pattern of relating to and perceiving the world is inflexible and maladaptive, it is described as a **personality disorder**.
- The pattern is enduring and crosses a broad range of social, occupational, and personal areas.
- The pattern can be traced back to adolescence or early adulthood and may affect cognition, affect, interpersonal functioning, or impulse control.

Cluster A Personality Disorders

- Cluster A disorders include the *paranoid personality disorder, schizoid personality, and schizotypal personality disorders.*
- This cluster includes the distrustful, emotionally detached, eccentric personalities.

Cluster B Personality Disorders

- Cluster B disorders include the *antisocial personality disorders, borderline, histrionic, and narcissistic personality disorders.*
- This cluster includes those who have disregard for others, with unstable and intense interpersonal relationships, excessive attention seeking, and entitlement issues with a lack of empathy for others.

Cluster C Personality Disorders

- Cluster C personality disorders include the avoidant personality, dependent personality, and the obsessive-compulsive personality disorders.
- This cluster includes the avoider of social situations; the clinging, submissive personality; and the person preoccupied with details, rules, and order. (APA 2000)

CLINICAL PEARL – Obsessive-Compulsive Personality Disorder (OCPD) is often confused with Obsessive-Compulsive Disorder (OCD). OCD is an *anxiety disorder* that is *ego-dystonic* (uncomfortable to person), whereas OCPD is a rigid way of functioning in the world. OCD clients want to change and dislike their disorder, whereas OCPD clients do not see that there is any problem with their excessive detail or controlling ways. They do not see that they need to change.

Borderline Personality Disorder (BPD)

Signs & Symptoms	Cause	Rule Outs	Labs/Tests/Exams	Interventions
• Pattern of unstable interpersonal relationships • Fear of abandonment • Splitting: Idealize and devalue (love/hate) • Impulsive (2 areas: sex, substance abuse, binge eating, reckless driving) • Suicidal gestures/ self mutilation • Intense mood changes lasting a few hours • Chronic emptiness • Intense anger • Transient paranoid ideation	• Genetic predisposition • Family hx of mood disorders; may be a variant of/ related to bipolar disorder • Physical/ sexual abuse • About 2% of general population • Predominantly female (75%)	• Mood disorders (often co-occur) • Histrionic, schizotypal, paranoid, antisocial, dependent, and narcissistic PDs • Personality change due to a general medical condition	• Millon Clinical Multiaxial Inventory-III (MCMI-III) • Psychiatric evaluation • Mental status exam • BDI • CAGE • SMAST • Physical exam, routine lab work, TFT	• Linehan DBT (dialectical behavior therapy) • CBT • Group, individual, family therapy (long-term therapy) • Special strategies • Boundary setting • Be aware that these can be difficult clients even for experienced MH professionals • Pharmacotherapy: antidepressants, mood stabilizers, antipsychotics. Caution with benzodiazepines (dependence)

Client/Family Education: Personality Disorders

- Share personality disorder with client and family and educate about the disorder. In this way the client has a basis/framework to understand his/her recurrent patterns of behavior.
- Work with client and family in identifying most troublesome behaviors (temper tantrums) and work with client on alternative responses and to anticipate triggers.
- For clients who act out using suicidal gestures, an agreement may have to be prepared to help client work on impulse control. Agreement might set an amount of time that client will not mutilate and what client will do instead (call a friend/ therapist/listen to music). Need to teach alternative behaviors.
- It is better to lead clients to a conclusion ("Can you see why your friend was angry when you did such and such?") rather than telling the client what he or she did, especially those clients with a borderline personality disorder.
- Because these are long-standing, fixed views of the world, they require time and patience and can be frustrating to treat. Usually require an experienced therapist.
- Although borderline personality disorder receives a lot of attention, all clients with personality disorders (narcissists; dependent, avoidant personalities) suffer in relationships, occupations, social situations.
- Client needs to be willing to change, and a therapeutic (trusting) relationship is a prerequisite for anyone with a personality disorder to accept criticisms/frustrations. Some clients believe the problems rest with everyone but themselves.
- A helpful book for BPD clients and families to read in order to understand the borderline personality is: Kreisman JJ, Straus H: I Hate You – Don't Leave Me. New York, Avon Books, 1991.
- For professionals: Linehan MM: Skills Training Manual for Treating Borderline Personality Disorder. New York: Guilford Press, 1993.

Disorders of Childhood and Adolescence

Disorders diagnosed in childhood or adolescence include:

- **Mental retardation** – onset before age 18 and IQ < 70.
- **Learning disorders** – include mathematics, reading disorder, disorder of written expression, with academic functioning below age, education level, intelligence.
- **Communication disorders** – speech or language difficulties, including expressive language, mixed receptive-expressive language, phonological disorder, and stuttering.
- **Motor skills** – developmental coordination disorder, with poor motor coordination for age and intelligence.
- **Pervasive developmental disorders** – deficits in multiple developmental areas and include autism, Asperger's, Rett's, and childhood disintegrative disorder.
- **Feeding/eating disorders** – disturbances of infancy and childhood, including pica, rumination, and feeding disorder of infancy and early childhood.
- **Tic disorders** – vocal and motor tics such as Tourette's, transient tic, and chronic motor or vocal tic disorder.
- **Elimination disorders** – include encopresis and enuresis.
- **Attention deficit/disruptive behavior** – includes ADHD, predominantly inattentive, predominantly hyperactive-impulsive, or combined type; conduct disorder, oppositional defiant disorder, and others.
- **Others** – separation anxiety, selective mutism, reactive attachment disorder, and so forth. (APA 2000)

Mental Retardation

50 – 70 IQ MILD	Able to live independently with some assistance; some social skills; does well in structured environment
35 – 49 IQ MODERATE	Some independent functioning; needs to be supervised; some unskilled vocational abilities (workshop)
20 – 34 IQ SEVERE	Total supervision; some basic skills (simple repetitive tasks)
< 20 IQ PROFOUND	Total care and supervision; care is constant and continual; little to no speech/no social skills ability

Modified from Townsend 2005, with permission

Attention Deficit/Hyperactivity Disorder (ADHD)

- ADHD is characterized either by *persistent inattention* or by *hyperactivity/impulsivity* for at least 6 months.
- Inattention includes
  - Carelessness and inattention to detail
  - Cannot sustain attention and does not appear to be listening
  - Does not follow through on instructions and unable to finish tasks, chores, homework
  - Difficulty with organization and dislikes activities that require concentration and sustained effort
  - Loses things; distracted by extraneous stimuli; forgetful
- Hyperactivity-impulsivity includes
  - Hyperactivity
  - Fidgeting, moving feet, squirming
  - Leaves seat before excused
  - Runs about/climbs excessively
  - Difficulty playing quietly
  - "On the go" and "driven by motor"
  - Excessive talking
- Impulsivity
  - Blurts out answers, speaks before thinking
  - Problem waiting his/her turn
  - Interrupts or intrudes
- Impairment is present before age 7, and impairment is present in at least two settings (or more).
- Significant impairment in functioning in social, occupational, or academic setting. Symptoms are not caused by another disorder. Prevalence rate, school-aged children: 3 – 7%. (APA 2000)
- Many *possible* causes: genetics; biochemical (possible neurochemical deficits [dopamine, norepinephrine]); intrauterine exposure to substances such as alcohol or smoking; exposure to lead, dyes, and additives in food; stressful home environments.
- *Adult ADHD* – Study presented at American Psychiatric Association (May 2004) estimates about 2.9% of the US general adult population suffers from ADHD. (Faraone 2004)

Nonpharmacologic ADHD Treatments

- Individual/family therapy
- *Behavior modification:* clear expectations and limits
- Break commands up into clear steps
- Support desired behaviors and immediately respond to undesired behaviors with consequences
- *Natural consequences* helpful (loses bicycle; do not replace; has to save own money to replace)
- *Time outs* may be needed for cooling down/reflecting
- *Role-playing:* helpful in teaching friend-friend interactions; helps child prepare for interactions and understand how intrusive behaviors annoy and drive friends away
- *Inform school:* important that school knows about ADHD diagnosis, as this is a disability (Americans with Disabilities Act)
- Seek out special education services
- *Classroom:* sit near teacher, one assignment at a time, written instructions, untimed tests, tutoring (need to work closely with teacher and explain child's condition [ADHD])
- *Nutritional:* many theories remain controversial but include food sensitivities (Feingold diet, allergen elimination), leaky gut syndrome, Nambudripad's allergy elimination technique), supplementation (thiamine), minerals (magnesium, iron), essential fatty acids, amino acids; evaluate for lead poisoning

For Pharmacologic ADHD Treatments — *See Drug Tab.*

ADHD/Learning Disability Web Sites:

Internet Mental Health: ADHD
http://www.mentalhealth.com/dis/p20-ch01.html
National Institute of Mental Health: ADHD
http://gopher.nimh.nih.gov/healthinformation/adhdmenu.cfm
Children & Adults With ADHD (CHADD) http://www.chadd.org/
National Center for Learning Disabilities http://www.ld.org/

Conduct Disorder/Oppositional Defiant Disorder

■ *Conduct disorder* (*CD*) (serious rule violation, aggression, destruction) and *oppositional defiant disorder* (*ODD*) (negative, hostile, defiant) are other important disorders of childhood and adolescence.

■ Serious co-morbidities include CD/ADHD, ODD/ADHD, and CD/ADHD/GAD/MDD.

■ A position paper by the International Society of Psychiatric-Mental Health Nurses, entitled *Prevention of Youth Violence*, can be found at: http://ispn-psych.org/docs/3-01-youth-violence.pdf

Because of size limitations, PsychNotes can provide only limited and basic information related to the unique and comprehensive specialty of child and adolescent psychiatry. For more complete coverage, refer to any of the standard psychiatric textbooks and references.

Psychiatric Interventions

Therapeutic Relationship/Alliance

- The *therapeutic relationship* is not concerned with the skills of the mental health professional but rather the attitudes and the relationship between the mental health professional and the client. This relationship comes out of the creation of a safe environment, conducive to communication and trust.
- An *alliance* is formed when the professional and the client are working together cooperatively in the best interest of the client. The therapeutic relationship begins the moment the mental health professional and client first meet (Shea 1999).

Core Elements of a Therapeutic Relationship

- *Communication/rapport* – It is important to establish a *connection* before a relationship can develop. Encouraging the client to speak, using open-ended questions, is helpful. Asking general (not personal) questions can relax the client in an initial session. It is important to project a *caring, nonjudgmental attitude.*
- *Trust* – A core element of a therapeutic relationship is trust. Many clients have experienced disappointment and unstable, even abusive relationships. Trust develops over time and remains part of the process. *Without trust, a therapeutic relationship is not possible.* Other important elements are *confidentiality, setting boundaries, consistency.*
- Dignity/Respect – Many clients have been abused and humiliated and have low self-esteem. If treated with dignity through the therapeutic relationship, clients can learn to regain their dignity.
- *Empathy* – Empathy is not sympathy (caught up in client's feelings) but is, rather, open to understanding the "client's perceptions" and helps the client understand these better through therapeutic exploration.
- *Genuineness* – In some way genuineness relates to trust because it says to the client: *I am honest and I am a real person.* Again, it will allow the client to get in touch with her/his "real" feelings and to learn from and grow from the relationship.

Therapeutic Use of Self

Ability to use one's own personality consciously and in full awareness to establish relatedness and to structure interventions (Travelbee 1971). Requires self awareness and self understanding.

Phases of Relationship Development

■ *Orientation phase* – This is the phase where the mental health professional and client first meet and where initial impressions are formed.
  ◆ Rapport is established and trust begins.
  ◆ The relationship and the connection are most important.
  ◆ Client is encouraged to identify the problem(s) and become a collaborative partner in helping him/herself.
  ◆ Once rapport and a connection are established, the relationship is ready for the next phase.

■ *Identification phase* – In this phase the mental health professional and client are
  ◆ Clarifying perceptions and setting expectations, in and for the relationship.
  ◆ Getting to know and understand each other.

■ *Exploitation (working) phase* – The client is committed to the process and is involved in the relationship and takes responsibility and shows some independence.
  ◆ This is also known as the *working phase*, because this is where the hard work begins.
  ◆ Client must believe and know that the mental health professional is caring and on his/her side when dealing with the more difficult issues during therapeutic exploration.
  ◆ If this phase is entered too early, before trust is developed, clients may suddenly terminate if presented with painful information.

■ *Resolution phase* – The client has gained all that he/she needs from the relationship and is ready to leave.
  ◆ This may involve having met stated goals or resolution of a crisis.
  ◆ Be aware of fear of abandonment and need for closure.
  ◆ Both mental health professional and client may experience sadness, which is normal.

◆ Dependent personalities may need help with termination, reflecting upon the positives and the growth that has taken place through the relationship. (Peplau 1992)

■ If a situation brings a client back for therapy, the relationship has already been established (trust); therefore, *there is not a return to the orientation phase.* However, both will 1) identify new issues and 2) re-establish expectations of proposed outcomes. It will now be *easier to move into the working phase of the relationship,* and this will be done more quickly.

CLINICAL PEARL – *Trust* and *safety* are core elements of a therapeutic alliance, as many clients have experienced abuse, inconsistency, broken promises, and "walking on eggs."

Nonverbal Communication

Nonverbal communication may be a better indication of what is going on with a client than verbal explanations.

◆ Although verbal is important, it is only one component of an evaluation.
◆ Equally important to develop your skills of observation.
◆ Some clients are not in touch with their feelings, and only their behaviors (clenched fist, head down, arms crossed) will offer clues to feelings.
◆ Nonverbal communication may offer the client clues as to how the mental health professional is feeling, as well.

■ *Physical appearance* – A neat appearance is suggestive of someone who cares for him/herself and feels positive about self. Clients with schizophrenia or depression may appear disheveled and unkempt.
■ *Body movement/ posture* – Slow or rapid movements can suggest depression or mania; a slumped posture, depression. Medication-induced body movements and postures include: pseudoparkinsonism (antipsychotic); akathisia (restlessness/moving legs [antipsychotic]). Warmth (smiling) and coldness (crossed arms) are also nonverbally communicated.
■ *Touch* – Touch forms a bridge or connection to another. Touch has different meanings based on culture, and some cultures touch more than others. Touch can have a very positive effect, but touching requires permission to do so. Many psychiatric clients have had "boundary violations," and so an innocent touch may be misinterpreted.

Communication Techniques

Technique	Rationale	Example
Reflecting	Reflects back to clients their emotions, using their own words	C: John never helps with the housework. MHP: You're angry that John doesn't help.
Silence	Allows client to explore all thoughts/feelings; prevents cutting conversation at a critical point or missing something important	Professional nods with some local cues from time to time so client knows MHP is listening, but does not interject.
Paraphrasing	Restating using different words to assure you have understood the client; helps clarify	C: My grandkids are coming over today and I don't feel well. MHP: Your grandkids are coming over, but you wish they weren't, because you are not well. Is that what you are saying?

■ *Eyes* – The ability to maintain eye contact during conversation offers clues as to social skills and self esteem. Without eye contact, there is a "break in the connection" between two people. A lack of eye contact can suggest suspiciousness, something to hide. Remember cultural interpretations of eye contact. (See Basics Tab)

Voice – Voice can be a clue to the mood of a client. Pitch, loudness, and rate of speech are all important clues. Manic clients speak loudly, rapidly, and with pressured speech. Anxious clients may speak with a high pitch and rapidly. Depressed clients speak slowly, and obtaining information may feel like "pulling teeth."

Communication Techniques		
Technique	**Rationale**	**Example**
Making observations	Helps client recognize feelings he/she may not be aware of and connect with behaviors	MHP: *Every time we talk about your father you become very sad.*
Open-ended/ broad questions	Encourages client to take responsibility for direction of session; avoids yes/no responses	MHP: What would you like to deal with in this session?
Encourage-ment	Encourages client to continue	MHP: Tell me more... uh huh...and then?
Reframing	Presenting same information from another perspective (more positive)	C: I lost my keys, couldn't find the report, and barely made it in time to turn my report in. MHP: In spite of all that, *you did turn your report in.*
Challenging idea/belief system	Break through denial or fixed belief. Always done with a question.	MHP: Who told you that you were incompetent? Where did you get the idea that you can't say no?
Recognizing change/ recognition	Reinforces interest in client and positive reinforcement (this is not a compliment).	MHP: I noticed that you were able to start our session today rather than just sit there.
Clarification	Assures that MHP did not misunderstand; encourages further exploration.	MHP: This is what I thought you said...; is that correct?

(Continued on following page)

Communication Techniques (Continued)

Technique	Rationale	Example
Exploring in detail	If it appears a particular topic is important, then the MHP asks for more detail. MHP then takes the lead from the client (client may resist exploring further.)	MHP: This is the first time I've heard you talk about your sister; would you like to tell me more about her?
Focusing	Use when a client is covering multiple topics rapidly (bipolar/anxious) and speed help focusing.	A lot is going on, but let's discuss the issue of your job loss, as I would like to hear more about that.
Metaphors/ symbols	Sometimes clients speak to us in us in symbolic ways and need translation.	C: The sky is just so grey today and night comes so early now. MHP: Sounds like you are feeling somber.
Acceptance	Positive regard and open to communication	I hear what you are saying. Yes, uh-huh (full attention)

Therapeutic Milieu

- In the **therapeutic milieu** (*milieu* is French for surroundings or environment), the entire environment of the hospital is set up so that every action, function, and encounter is therapeutic.
- The therapeutic community is a smaller representation of the larger community/society outside.
- The coping skills and learned behaviors within the community will also translate to the larger community outside.

Seven Basic Assumptions:

1. The health in each individual is to be realized and encouraged to grow.
2. Every interaction is an opportunity for therapeutic intervention.
3. The client owns his or her own environment.
4. Each client owns his or her own behavior.
5. Peer pressure is a useful and powerful tool.
6. Inappropriate behaviors are dealt with as they occur.
7. Restrictions and punishment are to be avoided.

(Skinner 1979)

Group Interventions

Stages of Group Development

I. The Initial Stage (in/out)

- Leader orients the group and sets up the ground rules, including confidentiality.
- There may be confusion and questions about the purpose of the group.
- Members question themselves in relation to others and how they will fit in the group.

II. The Conflict Stage (top/bottom)

- Group is concerned with pecking order, role, and place in group.
- There can be criticism and judgment.
- Therapist may be criticized as group finds its way.

III. Cohesiveness (Working) Stage (near/far)

- After conflict comes a group spirit, and a bond and trust develop among the members.
- Concern is now with closeness, and an "us versus them" attitude develops: those in the group versus those *outside the group.*
- Eventually becomes a mature working group.

IV. Termination

- Difficult for long-term groups; discuss well before termination.
- There will be grieving and loss. (Yalom 1995)

Leadership Styles

◆ **Autocratic** – The autocratic leader essentially " rules the roost." He or she is the most important person of the team and has very strong opinions of how and when things should be done. Members of a group are not allowed to make independent decisions, as the autocrat trusts only his/her opinions. The autocrat is concerned with power and control and is very good at persuasion. High productivity/low morale.

◆ **Democratic** – The democratic leader focuses on the group and empowers the group to take responsibility and make decisions. Problem solving and taking action are important, along with offering alternative solutions to problems (by group members). Lower productivity/high morale.

◆ **Laissez-Faire** – This leaderless style results in confusion because of the lack of direction and noninvolvement; it also results in low productivity and morale. (Lippitt & White 1938)

Individual Roles/Difficult Group Members

■ **Monopolizer** – Involved in some way in every conversation, offering extensive detail, or always presents with a "crisis of the week" (minimizing anyone else's concerns/issues).

◆ *Always has experienced a similar situation:* I know what you mean, my dog died several years ago and it was so painful, and I am still not over it.

◆ Monopolizer will eventually cause anger and resentment in the group if leader does not control the situation; dropouts result.

■ **Help-rejecting complainer** – Requests help from the group and then rejects each and every possible solution, so as to demonstrate the hopelessness of the situation.

◆ No one else's situation is as bad as the help-rejecting complainer's. *(You think you have it bad, wait until you hear my story.)*

◆ Often looks to the group leader for advice and help and competes with others for this help, and because he/she is not happy, no one else can be happy either.

◆ Requires an experienced leader who does not try to save the client but accepts the client's stance of hopelessness, while using group cohesiveness to help client see patterns.

- **Silent client** – Does not participate but observes.
  - Could be fear of self-disclosure, exposing weaknesses. Possibly feels unsafe in leaderless group.
  - Some clients do gain from mere vicarious experience, but in general, participation is needed to benefit from a group.
  - Does not respond well to pressure or being put on the spot, but must somehow be respectfully included and addressed.
  - The long-term silent client does not benefit from being in a group, nor does the group, and should possibly withdraw from the group.
- **Boring client** – The boring client is "boring" – no spontaneity, no fun, no opinions, and a need to present to the world what the client believes the world wants to see and hear.
  - If you are bored by the client, likely the client is boring.
  - Requires the gradual removal of barriers that have kept the individual buried inside for years.
  - Often tolerated by others but seldom missed if leaves the group.
- **Narcissist** – Lack of awareness of others in the group to seeing others as mere appendages and existing for one's own end; feels special and not a part of the group (masses).
  - They expect from others but give nothing.
  - Can gain from some groups and leaders.
- **Psychotic client** – Should not be included in early formative stages of a group.
  - If a client who is a member of an established group decompensates, then the group can be supportive because of an earlier connection and knowledge of the nonpsychotic state of the person.
- **Borderline client** – Can be challenging in a group because of emotional volatility, unstable interpersonal relationships, fears of abandonment, anger control issues, to name a few.
  - Borderline clients idealize or devalue (splitting) – the leader is at first great and then awful.
  - Can be frustrating to group members and leader and very tiring.
  - Some borderline group members who connect with a group may be helped as trust develops and borderline client is able to accept some frustrations and mild criticisms. (Yalom 1995)

CLINICAL PEARL – It is important to understand that subgroups (splitting off of smaller group/unit) can and do develop within the larger group. Loyalty transferred to a subgroup undermines overall goals of larger group (some clients are in and some out). May be indirect hostility to leader. Some subgroups and extragroup activities are positive as long as there is not a splitting from/hostility toward larger group. Group needs to openly address feelings about subgroups and outside activities – if splintering or secretiveness continues, will be a detriment to group's cohesiveness and therapeutic benefit.

Yalom's Therapeutic Factors

The factors involved in and derived from group experience that help and are of value to group members and therapeutic success are:

- *Instillation of hope* – Hope that this group experience will be therapeutic and effective.
- *Universality* – Despite our uniqueness, there are common denominators that allow for a connection and reduce our feelings of being alone in our plight.
- *Didactic interaction* – In some instances, instruction and education can help us understand our circumstances, and such information relieves anxiety and offers power, such as understanding cancer, anxiety disorder, or HIV.
- *Direct advice* – In some groups, advice giving can be helpful when one has more experience and can truly help another (cancer survivor helping newly diagnosed cancer patient). Too much advice-giving can impede. Advice giving/talking/refusing tells much about the group members and stage of group.
- *Altruism* – Although altruism suggests a concern for others that is unselfish, it is learning that through giving to others, one truly receives. One can find meaning through giving.
- *Corrective recapitulation of the primary family group* – Many clients develop dysfunctions related to the primary group – *the family of origin*. There are often unresolved relationships, strong emotions, and unfinished business. The group often serves as an opportunity to work out some of these issues as leaders and group members remind each other of primary family members, even if not consciously.

- *Socializing techniques* – Either the direct or indirect learning of social skills. Helpful to those whose interpersonal relationships have fallen short because of poor social skills. Often provided by group feedback, such as *You always turn your body away from me when I talk and you seem bored.* In many instances, individuals are *unaware* of the behaviors that are disconcerting or annoying to others.
- *Imitative behavior* – Members may model other group members, which may help in exploring new behaviors.

Family Therapy

Family Therapy Models/Theories

- *Intergenerational* – The theory of *Murray Bowen* (1994) that says problems are multigenerational and pass down from generation to generation until addressed. *Requires direct discussion and clarification with previous generation members if possible.* Concerned with level of individual differentiation and anxiety, triangles, nuclear family emotional system, and multigenerational emotional process. Therapist must remain a neutral third party.
- *Contextual* – The therapy of *Boszormenyi-Nagy* that focuses on give and take between family members, entitlement and fulfillment, fairness, and the family ledger (an accounting of debits and merits).
- *Structural* – Developed by *Salvador Minuchin* and views the family as a social organization with a structure and distinct patterns. Therapist takes an active role and challenges the existing order.
- *Strategic* – Associated with *Jay Haley* and focuses on problem definition and resolution, using active intervention.
- *Communications* – Focuses on the communications in the family and emphasizes reciprocal affection and love; the *Satir model.*
- *Systemic* – Involves multidimensional thinking and use of paradox (tactics that appear opposite to therapy goals, but designed to achieve goals); also called the *Milan model.*

CLINICAL PEARL – In dealing with families, it is important to have an understanding of how families operate, whatever model is used. A model offers a framework for viewing the family. A family is a subsystem within a larger system (community/society) and will reflect the values and culture of that society. Unlike working with individuals, it is the *family that is the client.*

Genogram

A genogram is a visual diagram of a family over two or three generations. It provides an overview of the family and any significant emotional and medical issues and discord among members. It offers insight into patterns and unresolved issues/conflicts throughout the generations.

Common Genogram Symbols

KEY

Male □

Female ○

Married (m) —

Divorced (d) —|—

Separated(s) —/—

Unmarried relationship – –

Conflictual relationship ∿∿∿

Overclose relationship ⫽⫽⫽

Offspring |

Pregnant ▼

Miscarriage or abortion ▽

Adopted (boy) □

Twins (boys) ⊓ ⊓

Death ✕

NOTE: Include ages and dates of significant events when known.

Sample Genogram

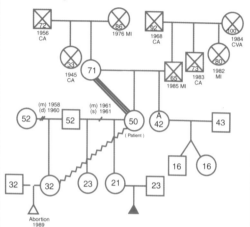

(From Townsend Essentials, 3/e, 2005, with permission.)

Cognitive Behavioral Therapy

- Cognitive behavioral therapy (CBT) deals with the relationship between cognition, emotion, and behavior.
  - Cognitive aspects are: automatic thoughts, assumptions, and distortions.
  - Individuals are often unaware of the *automatic thoughts* that may affect beliefs and behaviors, such as *I never do well in school* or *I am stupid.*
  - Deep-seated beliefs or "*schemas*" affect our perceptions of the world as well.
  - And finally, individuals are also influenced by *distortions* in their thinking.

■ Important aspects of CBT include agenda setting, review, feedback, and homework.

■ Some techniques may involve treating the behaviors rather than the cognitive aspects.

◆ Fearful, dysfunctional clients respond better to behavioral versus cognitive interventions. This may involve task or activity assignments.

◆ Other behavioral interventions are: social skills training, assertiveness training, deep-muscle relaxation, exposure and systematic desensitization techniques, and in vivo intervention (phobias/agoraphobia).

Distortions in Thinking

■ *Catastrophizing* – an uncomfortable event is turned into a catastrophe.

■ *Dichotomous thinking* – either/or thinking, such as I am all good or I am evil.

■ *Mind reading* – believes that the person knows what the other is thinking without clarifying.

■ *Selective abstraction* – focusing on one aspect rather than all aspects. Individual hears only the one negative comment during a critique and does not hear the five positive comments.

■ *Fortune telling* – anticipates a negative future event without facts or outcome. I know I am going to fail that test.

■ *Overgeneralization* – one event is now representative of the entire situation. A forgotten anniversary is interpreted as the marriage is over and will never be the same.

CLINICAL PEARL – CBT has been shown to be quite effective in treating depression and anxiety disorders (panic/phobia/OCD) and is very helpful when used in conjunction with medication. Through CBT, clients learn to change their thinking and to "reframe" their views/thoughts as well as learn tools/techniques to deal with future episodes. CBT provides the client with a sense of control over his/her fears, depression, and anxiety, as there is an active participation in treatment and outcome.

Complementary Therapies

- *Art therapy* – the use of art media, images, and the creative process to reflect human personality, interests, concerns, and conflicts. Very helpful with children and traumatic memories.
- *Biofeedback* – learned control of the body's physiological responses either voluntarily (muscles) or involuntarily (autonomic nervous system), such as the control of blood pressure or heart rate.
- *Dance therapy* – as the mind/body is connected, dance therapy focuses on direct expression of emotion through the body, affecting feelings, thoughts, and the physical and behavioral responses.
- *Guided imagery* – imagination is used to visualize improved health; has positive effect on physiological responses.
- *Meditation* – self-directed relaxation of body and mind; health-producing benefits through stress reduction.
- *Others:* humor therapy, deep-muscle relaxation, prayer, acupressure, Rolfing, pet therapy, massage therapy, and so forth.

CLINICAL PEARL – Never underestimate the benefit of the complementary therapies. Complementary is often referred to as alternative therapy. In some ways, alternative is a misnomer because these are not alternatives but should be complements to traditional treatments. Both go hand in hand in a comprehensive approach to healing and treatment of the body, mind, and spiritual self.

Psychotropic Drugs

Over 50 *psychotropic drug monographs* can be found and printed out at: http://www.fadavis.com/psychnotes/

Psychopharmacologic Agents

Antianxiety (Anxiolytic) Agents
Used in the treatment of generalized anxiety, OCD, panic disorder, PTSD, phobic disorders, insomnia, and others and include benzodiazepines (alprazolam), azaspirones (buspirone), alpha-2 adrenergics (clonidine), antihistamines (hydroxyzine), beta-blockers (propranolol), antidepressants (doxepin), and hypnosedatives for insomnia, such as barbiturates (phenobarbital) and imidazopyridine (zolpidem).

Antidepressants
Used in the treatment of depression, bipolar (depressed), OCD, and others and include the tricyclics (doxepin, imipramine), MAOIs (phenelzine), SSRIs (fluoxetine, sertraline), SNRIs (venlafaxine), and others (bupropion [Wellbutrin], trazodone [Desyrel]).

Mood Stabilizers
Used in the treatment of bipolar disorder (mania/depression), aggression, schizoaffective, and others, and include lithium, anticonvulsants (valproic acid, carbamazepine, lamotrigine), calcium channel blockers (verapamil), alpha-2 adrenergics (clonidine), and beta-adrenergics (propranolol).

Antipsychotic (Neuroleptic) Agents
Used in the treatment of schizophrenia, psychotic episodes (depression/organic [dementia]/substance induced), bipolar disorder, agitation, delusional disorder, and others, and include the phenothiazines (chlorpromazine, thioridazine), butyrophenones (haloperidol), thioxanthenes (thiothixene), diphenylbutyl piperidines (pimozide), dibenzoxazepine (loxapine), dihydroindolone (molindone), dibenzodiazepine (clozapine), benzisoxazole (risperidone), thienobenzodiazepine (olanzapine), benzothiazolyl piperazine (ziprasidone), and dihydrocarbostyril (aripiprazole).
Although other agents (e.g., stimulants) may be used in the treatment of psychiatric disorders, the most common therapeutic classes and agents are listed above.

For a detailed listing of over 50 psychotropic monographs, which can be printed, log onto: http://www.fadavis.com/psychnotes/

Psychotropic Drug Tables that follow include half life (T$^1/_2$); Canadian drug trade names (*in italics*), most frequent side effects (<u>underlined</u>), and life threatening side effects (ALL CAPS).

Antianxiety (Anxiolytic) Agents

Benzodiazepines

Generic Name	Trade Name	Adult Dose Range	Common Side Effects	CAUTION
Alprazolam Intermediate T½: 12–15 h	Xanax Xanax XR Apo-Alpraz Novo-Alprazol Nu-Alpraz	0.75–4 mg/d; not to exceed 10 mg/d Xanax XR for panic disorder (usual range, 3–6 mg/d) Use: Anxiety, panic disorder	<u>Dizziness, drowsiness, lethargy,</u> headache, blurred vision, constipation, diarrhea. Possible physical/ psychological dependence, tolerance, paradoxical excitation	Hepatic dysfunction *Contraindicated:* pregnancy/lactation; narrow-angle glaucoma; concurrent ketoconazole or itraconazole; ↓ *dose* elderly/debilitated.
Lorazepam Intermediate T½: 10–20 h	Ativan Apo-Lorazepam Novo-Lorazem Nu-Loraz	2–6 mg/d (up to 10 mg/d) insomnia: 2–4 mg/h Use: Anxiety/ insomnia/ seizures	Same as alprazolam Rapid IV only: APNEA, CARDIAC ARREST	*Contraindicated:* pregnancy/lactation; narrow-angle glaucoma. *Caution:* severe hepatic/renal/ pulmonary impairment; ↓ *dose* elderly/debilitated.

			Benzodiazepines	
Generic Name	**Trade Name**	**Adult Dose Range**	**Common Side Effects**	**CAUTION**
Clonazepam Long T½: 18–50 h	Klonopin Rivotril Syn-Clonaze-pam	1.5–4 mg/d (panic/anxiety); as high as 6 mg/d: up to 20 mg/d for seizures Use: Panic disorder, seizure disorders	<u>Drowsiness, behavioral changes,</u> ataxia, abnormal eye movements, palpitations Possible physical/psychological dependence, tolerance	*Contraindicated:* severe liver disease. *Caution:* pregnancy/lactation/children; narrow-angle glaucoma; chronic respiratory disease, porphyria.
Oxazepam Intermediate T½: 5–15 h	Serax Apo-Oxazepam Novoxazam	30–120 mg/d (anxiety) 45–120 mg/d (sedative/hypnotic/alcohol mgmt) Use: Anxiety, alcohol withdrawal, insomnia	<u>Dizziness, drowsiness,</u> blurred vision, tachycardia, constipation. Possible physical/psychological dependence, tolerance, etc.	*Contraindicated:* pregnancy/lactation; narrow-angle glaucoma; *caution* in hepatic impairment and severe COPD; ↓ dose elderly/debilitated.

Antidepressants

Tricyclics

Generic Name	Trade Name	Adult Dose Range	Common Side Effects	CAUTION
Amitriptyline $T^1/_2 = 10$–50 h	Elavil Endep Apo- *Amitriptyline* Levate *Novotriptyn*	50–300 mg/d Use: Depression/ chronic pain	Lethargy, sedation, blurred vision, dry eyes, dry mouth, hypotension, constipation, ↑ appetite, weight gain, gynecomastia, ARRHYTHMIAS	*Contraindicated:* narrow-angle glaucoma/pregnancy/lactation. *Caution:* elderly; pre-existing CV disease, hx seizures, BPH.
Doxepin $T^1/_2 = 8$–25 h	Sinequan *Triadapin*	25–300 mg/d	Same as amitriptyline	Same as amitriptyline; *contraindicated:* post MI.
Desipramine $T^1/_2 = 12$–27 h	Norpramin *Pertofrane*	25–300 mg/d	Same as amitriptyline	Same as amitriptyline.
Imipramine $T^1/_2 = 8$–16 h	Tofranil Tofranil PM Apo- *Imipramine*	30–300 mg/d	Same as amitriptyline	Same as amitriptyline.

	Generic Name	Trade Name	Adult Dose Range	Common Side Effects	CAUTION
Selective Serotonin Reuptake Inhibitors (SSRIs)					
T¹/₂ = 1-3 d (norfluoxetine: 5-7 d)	Fluoxetine	Prozac Prozac weekly Sarafem	20 mg/d OCD: May require up to/not to exceed 80 mg/d _Prozac weekly:_ 90 mg/week (start 7 d after last 20-mg dose) Use: Depression, OCD, bulimia nervosa, panic disorder; Sarafem (for PMDD)	Anxiety, drowsiness, headache, insomnia, nervousness, diarrhea, sexual dysfunction, sweating, pruritus, tremor, flushing, myalgia, flulike syndrome, abnormal taste, weight loss, etc.	Serious fatal reaction with MAOIs Do not use with St. John's wort or SAMe Highly protein binding; drug-drug interactions with other P-450 system drugs. _Caution:_ hepatic/ renal/ pregnancy/lactation/ seizures.
T¹/₂ = 21 h	Paroxetine	Paxil Paxil CR	10-60 mg/d; CR: 12.5-75 mg/d Use: Depression, social anxiety/ panic, OCD, GAD, PTSD	Anxiety, drowsiness, insomnia, nausea, diarrhea, ejaculatory disturbance, sweating, etc.	Same as fluoxetine; **FDA warning:** do not prescribe to child/teen ≤ 18 y; assess for suicide; self injury. Caution: withdrawal syndrome

(Continued on following page)

Selective Serotonin Reuptake Inhibitors (SSRIs) (Continued)

Generic Name	Trade Name	Adult Dose Range	Common Side Effects	CAUTION
Sertraline $T^1/_2$ = 24 h	Zoloft	50–200 mg/d Use: Depression, panic disorder, OCD, PTSD, social anxiety disorder, PMDD	Drowsiness, dizziness, headache, fatigue, insomnia, nausea, diarrhea, dry mouth, sexual dysfunction, sweating, tremor, myalgia, anxiety, altered taste, hot flashes, etc.	Serious fatal reaction with MAOIs; concurrent pimozide; do not use with St. John's wort or SAMe; drug-drug interactions with drugs that inhibit the P-450 system. Caution: hepatic/renal/pregnancy/lactation/children.
Fluvoxamine $T^1/_2$ = 16 h	Luvox Apo-Fluvoxamine	50–300 mg/d Use: OCD (depression)	Headache, fatigue, insomnia, nervousness, nausea, diarrhea, decreased libido, anorgasmia, sweating, etc.	Same as sertraline.

Serotonin-Norepinephrine Reuptake Inhibitors (SNRIs)

Generic Name	Trade Name	Adult Dose Range	Common Side Effects	CAUTION
Venlafaxine $T^1/_2$ = 3–5 h; O-desmethylven-lafaxine (ODV) 9–11 h	Effexor Effexor XR	75–225 mg/d; XR: 75 mg/d; ↑ at 4-d intervals to recommended max of 225 mg/d (not to exceed 375 mg/d [severe inpatient depression]) Use: Depression; major depression; GAD and social anxiety disorder (XR only)	Anxiety, abnormal dreams, dizziness, hypertension; insomnia, nervousness, visual disturbances, hepatic/renal impairment/ seizures/ pregnancy/ lactation/ children ≤ 18 y.	Contraindication: MAOIs. Caution: CV disease & hypertension; Monitor blood pressure (systolic hypertension)
Nefazodone $T^1/_2$ = 2.4 h; hydroxynefaz-odone 1.5–4 h	Serzone*	200–600 mg/d Use: Major depression	anorexia, dry mouth, weight loss, sexual dysfunction, ecchymoses (bruising), Insomnia, dizziness, drowsiness, HEPATIC FAILURE; HEPATIC TOXICITY SEIZURES	Monitor LFTs; generic still available. Caution: Same as venlafaxine.

*Serzone voluntarily withdrawn from US/Canadian market & others

Others (Aminoketone/Triazolopyridine)

Generic Name	Trade Name	Adult Dose Range	Common Side Effects	CAUTION
Bupropion $T^1/_2 = 14$ h; metabolites may be longer	Wellbutrin Wellbutrin SR (twice daily dosing) Wellbutrin XL (once daily dosing) Zyban SR (smoking)	200–450 mg/d; not to exceed 450 mg/d (smoking not to exceed 300 mg/d) Use: Depression, ADHD (adults [unlabeled: SR only]); ↑ sexual desire (females); smoking (Zyban)	<u>Agitation</u>, <u>headache, dry mouth, nausea, vomiting, tremor</u>, weight gain or loss, SIADH, etc.	Risk: seizure disorder. Seizure risk increased at dose > 450 mg; avoid alcohol.Contraindicated: concurrent use MAOIs, hx eating disorders. Caution: renal/ hepatic/recent MI/geriatric/ pregnancy/ lactation/children.
Trazodone $T^1/_2 = 5$–9 h	Desyrel	150–400 mg/d (up to 600 mg/d inpatient) Use: Major depression; insomnia	<u>Drowsiness</u>, <u>hypotension</u>, <u>dry mouth</u>, blurred vision, priapism, impotence	Priapism (prolonged erection in males) medical emergency. Seek immediate care.

Monoamine Oxidase Inhibitors (MAOIs)

Generic Name	Trade Name	Adult Dose Range	Common Side Effects	CAUTION
Phenelzine T½ = Unknown	Nardil	45–90 mg/d Use: Atypical depression, panic disorder; other Rx ineffective or not tolerated	<u>Dizziness, headaches, insomnia, restlessness, blurred vision, arrythmias, orthostatic hypotension, diarrhea</u> **SEIZURES, HYPERTENSIVE CRISIS**	*Tyramine-free diet.* *Contraindicated:* liver/renal/ cerebrovascular disease/concurrent SSRIs/ antidepressants/ meperidine; pheochromocytoma, CHF. hx headache. *Caution:* CV disease, hyperthyroidism, seizures, geriatric patients, pregnancy, lactation, children. *Monitor BP and pulse.*
Tranylcypromine T½ = Unknown	Parnate	30–60 mg/d (max: 60 mg/d)	Same as phenelzine	Same as phenelzine.

Mood Stabilizers

Lithium/Anticonvulsants

Generic Name	Trade Name	Adult Dose Range	Common Side Effects	CAUTION
Lithium (Li) $T^{1}/_2 = 20–27$ h	Eskalith Eskalith CR Lithane Lithobid Lithonate Lithotabs *Carbolith* *Duralith*	Acute mania: 1800–2400 mg/d Maintenance: 300–1200 mg/d Use: Bipolar, acute mania & prophylaxis; depression prophylaxis	<u>Fatigue, headache, impaired memory</u>, ECG changes, <u>bloating, diarrhea, nausea, abdominal pain, polyuria, acne, hypothyroidism, tremors,</u> SEIZURES, ARRHYTHMIAS	Narrow therapeutic range (0.6–1.2 mEq/L). Need serum tests. Li ↓thyroid/renal function tests. Encephalopathy with haloperidol. *Contraindication:* pregnancy (teratogenicity).
Valproates divalproex sodium; valproic acid (VA) $T^{1}/_2 = 5–20$ h	Depakote, Depakote ER *Epival,* *Depacon,* *Depakene*	500–1500 mg/d (divalproex) ↑ to achieve effect/ plasma concentration Use: Bipolar, acute mania & prophylaxis	<u>Nausea, vomiting, indigestion,</u> sedation, rash, hyper-salivation, pancreatitis, weight gain, hyperammonemia (D/C VA). HEPATOTOXICITY	Liver/renal disease; bleeding disorders. LFTs; platelet/ coagulation tests, teratogenicity; need VA test (50–100 mcg/mL).

Anticonvulsants

Generic Name	Trade Name	Adult Dose Range	Common Side Effects	CAUTION
Carbamazepine (CBZ) $T^{1}/_{2}$ = initial: 18–55 h; long-term dosing: 12–17 h	Tegretol Tegretol-XR Teril Epitol Carbatrol Apo- *Carbamazepine* *Novo-Carbamaz* *Tegretol CR*	400–1200 mg/d (mania) Use: Bipolar: acute mania; mixed; seizures, trigeminal pain	Ataxia, drowsiness, blurred vision. APLASTIC ANEMIA, AGRANULO-CYTOSIS, THROMBOCY-TOPENIA, STEVENS-JOHNSON SYNDROME (SJS)	*Therapeutic Range* (4–12 µg/mL) Weekly CBC, platelet & reticulocyte counts, LFTs; impaired renal/liver/cardiac functions. *Sx of SJS:* cough, FUO, mucosal lesions, rash; stop CBZ.
Lamotrigine (LTG) $T^{1}/_{2}$ = 24 h	Lamictal	75–250 mg/d Use: Bipolar disorder, maintenance, especially depressive; seizures	Nausea, vomiting, dizziness, headache, ataxia photosensitivity, rash, STEVENS-JOHNSON SYN-DROME (SJS)	Assess for skin rash. If rash develops, stop LTG & contact MD; impaired renal/liver/cardiac functions.

Antipsychotics (Treatment of Bipolar Disorder)

Generic Name	Trade Name	Adult Dose Range	Common Side Effects	CAUTION
Olanzapine Olanzapine for injection $T^{1}/_{2} = 21$–54 h	Zyprexa Zyprexa IntraMuscular Zyprexa Zydis	10–20 mg/d Use: Bipolar: acute mania/ mixed episodes use alone or in combination; olanzapine + Li or + VA or + fluoxetine **IM:** 10 mg, bipolar mania agitation	Agitation, dizziness, headache, restlessness, sedation, orthostatic hypotension, constipation, dry mouth, weight gain, tremor; NMS; SEIZURES	Treatment-emergent diabetes. *Labs:* FBS, HgbA1c, lipids (esp. family hx diabetes, obesity); BMI. *Caution:* hepatic/ cardiovascular/ cerebrovascular/ seizures/BPH/ pregnancy/children.
Risperidone $T^{1}/_{2} = 3$ h (metabolite 21 h)	Risperdal Risperdal M-TAB	4–12 mg/d (>6 mg ↑ risk of EPS); ≥10 mg, EPS = haloperidol Use: Bipolar disorder, acute/ mixed; short term	EPS (akathisia), dizziness, aggression, insomnia, dry mouth, ↓ libido, weight gain/ loss, hyperprolactinemia, etc.; NMS, SEIZURES	Same as olanzapine; **cerebrovascular adverse event** in elderly w/dementia.

	Antipsychotic (Neuroleptic) Agents

Conventional Agents (Phenothiazines/Butyrophenones)

Generic Name	Trade Name	Adult Dose Range	Common Side Effects	CAUTION
Chlorpromazine (CPZ) T¹/₂ = initial 2 h; end 30 h	Thorazine Thor-Prom Apo-Chlorpromany Largactil Novo-Chlorpromazine	40–800 mg/d Use: Psychosis; combativeness **IM:** 25–50 mg: gradual ↑ to 300– 800 mg/d (IM: Significant hypotension)	Hypotension, (esp. par-enteral), sedation, blurred vision, dry eyes, constipation, dry mouth, photosen-sitivity, EPS, pseudo-parkinsonism, acute dystonia, TD, NMS, AGRANULOCYTOSIS	Seizure disorders, Parkinson's. Contraindications: glaucoma, myasthenia gravis, bone marrow depression, Addison's disease. Caution: geriatrics, BPH, pregnancy/lactation.
Haloperidol T¹/₂ = 21–24 h	Haldol Haldol Decanoate (HD) Apo-Haloperidol Haldol LA Novo-Peridol Peridol PMS Haloperidol	1–100 mg/d; **IM:** HD – 10–15 X daily dose Use: Psychotic disorders, schizophrenia, mania, drug-induced psychosis	EPS, blurred vision, constipation, dry mouth/eyes, galactorrhea, hypotension, drowsiness, TD, NMS, SEIZURES	Same as CPZ. Encephalopathy with lithium.

Atypical Agents (Dibenzodiazepine/Benzisoxazole)

Generic Name	Trade Name	Adult Dose Range	Common Side Effects	CAUTION
Clozapine $T^{1}/_{2}$ = 8–12 h	Clozaril	300–450 mg/d Not to exceed 900 mg/d Use: Refractory schizophrenia (unresponsive to other treatments)	<u>Dizziness, sedation, hypotension, tachycardia</u>, constipation, NMS, SEIZURES, AGRANULOCYTO-SIS, LEUKOPENIA, MYOCARDITIS (d/c clozapine)	Clozaril protocol: BP/pulse, monitor CBC (WBC/diff < 3000/mm^3 – withhold clozapine). *Caution:* CV/ hepatic/renal disease/seizure/ children.
Risperidone $T^{1}/_{2}$ = 3 h (metabolite 21 h)	Risperdal Risperdal M-TAB	4–12 mg/d (>6 mg ↑ risk of EPS); ≥10 mg, EPS = haloperidol Use: Schizophrenia, bipolar, acute/mixed	<u>Akathisia, dizziness, aggression</u>, insomnia, dry mouth, weight gain/loss, libido, hyperprolactin-emia, NMS	Treatment-emergent diabetes (see olanzapine); cerebrovascular AE (stroke) in elderly w/dementia.

		Atypical Agents (Thienobenzodiazepine/Dihydrocarbostyril)			
Generic Name	**Trade Name**	**Adult Dose Range**	**Common Side Effects**	**CAUTION**
Olanzapine **Olanzapine for injection** $T^1/_2 = 21-54$ h	Zyprexa Zyprexa IntraMuscular Zyprexa Zydis	5–20 mg/d Use: Schizophrenia, psychotic disorders, acute mania (anorexia nervosa) **IM: 10 mg, bipolar/ schizophrenia agitation**	Agitation, dizziness, sedation, orthostatic hypotension, constipation, dry mouth, weight gain, obesity; NMS, SEIZURES	Treatment-emergent diabetes. Labs: FBS, HgbA1c, lipids (esp. family hx diabetes, obesity); BMI. Caution: hepatic/ cardiovascular/ cerebrovascular/ seizures/BPH/ pregnancy/ children.
Aripiprazole $T^1/_2 = 75$ h (metabolite 94 h)	Abilify	10–30 mg/d Use: Schizophrenia **Oct. 2004: FDA approved: acute bipolar mania & mixed episodes**	Headache, nausea, anxiety, insomnia, orthostatic hypotension, ↑ salivation, ecchymoses, NMS	Seizure disorder, Alzheimer's dementia Treatment-emergent diabetes (see olanzapine).

Attention Deficit Hyperactivity Disorder (ADHD) Agents

Chemical Class	Generic/Trade	Dosage Range/Day
Amphetamines	Dextroamphetamine (Dexedrine; DextroStat)	5–40 mg
	Methamphetamine (Desoxyn)	5–25 mg
	Amphetamine mixtures (Adderall; Adderall XR*)	5–40 mg (XR: 10–30 mg)
Miscellaneous	Methylphenidate (Ritalin)	10–60 mg
	Pemoline (Cylert)	375–112.5 mg
	Atomoxetine (Strattera)	> 70 kg: 40–100 mg; ≤ 70 kg: 0.5–1.4 mg/kg
	Bupropion (Wellbutrin)	3 mg/kg

*Withdrawn from Canadian market.

From Townsend, 2005, p. 176, used with permission.

Cytochrome P-450, Half Life, and Protein Binding

The Cytochrome P-450 Enzyme System is involved in drug biotransformation and metabolism. It is important to develop a knowledge of this system to understand drug metabolism and especially drug interactions. Over 30 P-450 isoenzymes have been identified. The major isoenzymes include CYP1A2/2A6/2B6/2C8/2C9/2C19/2D6/2E1/3A4/3A5-7

Half Life is the time (hours) that it takes for 50% of a drug to be eliminated from the body. Time to total elimination involves halving the remaining 50%, and so forth, until total elimination. Half life is considered in determining frequency and in determining time to steady state, and the rule of thumb for **steady state** (stable concentration) **attainment** is 4 – 5 half lives. Because of fluoxetine's long half life, a 5-week washout is recommended after stopping fluoxetine and before starting an MAOI, to avoid a serious and possibly fatal reaction.

Protein Binding is the amount of drug that binds to the blood's plasma proteins; remainder circulates unbound. It is important to understand this concept when prescribing two or more highly protein-bound drugs, as one drug may be displaced, causing increased blood levels and adverse effects.

MAOI Diet (Tyramine) Restrictions

FOODS: MUST AVOID COMPLETELY

- Aged red wines (cabernet sauvignon/merlot/Chianti)
- Aged (smoked, aged, pickled, fermented, marinated, and processed) meats (pepperoni/bologna/salami, pickled herring, liver, frankfurters, bacon, ham)
- Aged/mature cheeses (blue/cheddar/provolone/Brie/Romano/Parmesan/Swiss)
- Overripe fruits and vegetables (overripe bananas/sauerkraut/all overripe fruit)
- Beans (fava/Italian/Chinese pea pod/fermented bean curd/soya sauce/tofu/miso soup)
- Condiments (bouillon cubes/meat tenderizers/canned soups/gravy/sauces/soy sauce)
- Soups (prepared/canned/ frozen)
- Beverages (beer/ales/vermouth/whiskey/liqueurs/nonalcoholic wines and beers)

FOODS: USE WITH CAUTION (MODERATION)

- Avocados (not overripe)
- Raspberries (small amounts)
- Chocolate (small amount)
- Caffeine (2– 8 oz. servings per day or less)
- Dairy products (limit to buttermilk, yogurt, and sour cream [small amounts]; cream cheese, cottage cheese, milk OK if fresh)

MEDICATIONS: MUST AVOID

- Stimulants and decongestants
- OTC medications (check with PCP/pharmacist)
- Opioids (e.g., meperidine)

(Continued on following page)

♦ Ephedrine/epinephrine
♦ Methyldopa
♦ Herbal remedies

Any questions about the above should be discussed with the psychiatrist, pharmacist, PCP or advanced practice nurse.

Medications and the Elderly (Start Low, Go Slow)

■ Relevant drug guides provide data about dosing for the elderly and debilitated clients.

■ The elderly (or debilitated clients) are started at lower doses, often half the recommended adult dose. This is due to:
  ♦ decreases in GI absorption
  ♦ a decrease in total body water (decreased plasma volume)
  ♦ decreased lean muscle and increased adipose tissue
  ♦ reduced first-pass effect in the liver and cardiac output
  ♦ decreased serum albumin
  ♦ decreased glomerular filtration and renal tubular secretion
  ♦ time to steady state is prolonged.

Because of decrease in lean muscle mass and increase in fat (retains lipophilic drugs [fat storing]), reduced first-pass metabolism, and decreased renal function, drugs may remain in the body longer and produce an additive effect.

ALERT: With the elderly, start doses low and titrate slowly. Drugs that result in postural hypotension, confusion, or sedation should be used cautiously or not at all in the elderly.

■ **Poor Drug Choices for the Elderly** – Drugs that cause postural hypotension or anticholinergic side effects (sedation):
  ♦ *TCAs* – anticholinergic (confusion, constipation, visual blurring); cardiac (conduction delay; tachycardia); alpha-1 adrenergic (orthostatic hypotension [falls]).
  ♦ *Benzodiazepines* – the shorter the half life, the greater the risk of falls. Choose a shorter half life. Lorazepam ($T_{1/2}$, 12 – 15 h) is a better choice than diazepam ($T_{1/2}$, 20 – 70 h; metabolites, up to 200 h).
  ♦ *Lithium* – use cautiously in elderly, especially if debilitated. Consider age, weight, mental state, and medical disorders and compare to side effect profile in selecting medications.

Antidepressants in Childhood & Adolescence (SSRIs)

ALERT: Childhood depression has been on the rise in the United States, coupled with an increase in the prescribing of antidepressants for adolescents and also children under age 5. The FDA has asked drug manufacturers of SSRIs to strengthen their warnings on package inserts and to observe for suicidal thinking and behaviors.

On June 10, 2003, the UK issued a warning that Seroxat (Paxil) must be not be used to treat depression in children under age 18, because of potential suicidal behavior. The Committee on Safety of Medicines said that the benefits of Seroxat did not outweigh the risks. The United States and Canada then followed suit. **Clearly, all children treated with SSRIs, as well as adults, need to be closely monitored and assessed for suicidal ideation and risk.** (Johnson 2003; Seroxat 2004; Health Canada 2004)

Neuroleptic Malignant Syndrome (NMS)

A serious and potentially fatal syndrome caused by antipsychotics and other drugs that block dopamine receptors. Important not to allow client to become *dehydrated* (predisposing factor). More common in warm climates, in summer. Possible genetic predisposition.

Signs and Symptoms
■ Fever: 103° – 105° F or greater
■ BP lability (hypertension or hypotension)
■ Tachycardia (>130 bpm)
■ Tachypnea (>25 rpm)
■ Agitation (respiratory distress, tachycardia)
■ Diaphoresis, pallor
■ Muscle rigidity (arm/abdomen like a board)
■ Change in mental status (stupor to coma)

Stop antipsychotic immediately
ALERT: NMS is a medical emergency (10% mortality rate); hospitalization needed. Lab test: Creatine kinase (CK) to determine injury to the muscle. Drugs used to treat NMS include: bromocriptine, dantroline, levodopa, lorazepam.

Antipsychotic Use Contraindications

■ Addison's disease
■ Bone marrow depression
■ Glaucoma (narrow-angle)
■ Myasthenia gravis

Antipsychotic-Induced Movement Disorders

Extrapyramidal Symptoms (EPS)

EPS are caused by antipsychotic treatment and need to be monitored/evaluated for early intervention.

■ Akinesia – rigidity and bradykinesia.
■ Akathisia – restlessness; movement of body; unable to keep still; movement of feet (do not confuse with anxiety).
■ Dystonia – spasmodic and painful spasm of muscle [torticollis (head pulled to one side); oculogyric [eyes roll to back of head]
■ Oculogyric crisis – eyes roll toward back of head. **This is an emergency situation.**
■ Pseudoparkinsonism – simulates Parkinson's disease with shuffling gait, drooling, muscular rigidity, and tremor.
■ Rabbit syndrome – rapid movement of the lips that simulate a rabbit's mouth movements.

Tardive Dyskinesia

Permanent dysfunction of voluntary muscles. Affects the mouth – tongue protrudes, smacking of lips, mouth movements; also choreoathetoid extremity movements.

ALERT: Evaluate clients on antipsychotics for possible tardive dyskinesia by using the Abnormal Involuntary Movement Scale (AIMS). (See AIMS form in Assessment Tab.)

Serotonin Syndrome

Can occur if client is taking one or more serotonergic drugs (e.g., SSRIs), especially higher doses. Do not combine SSRIs/SNRIs/clomipramine with MAOI; also, tryptophan, dextromethorphan combined with MAOI can produce this syndrome.

If stopping fluoxetine (long half life) to start an MAOI – must allow a 5-week wash-out period. At least 2 weeks for other SSRIs before starting an MAOI. Discontinue MAOI for 2 weeks before starting another antidepressant or other interacting drug.

Signs and Symptoms

- Change in mental status, agitation, confusion, restlessness, flushing
- Diaphoresis, diarrhea, lethargy
- Myoclonus (muscle twitching or jerks), tremors

If serotonergic medication is not discontinued, progresses to:

- Worsening myoclonus, hypertension, rigor
- Acidosis, respiratory failure, rhabdomyolysis

ALERT: Must discontinue serotonergic drug immediately. Emergency medical treatment and hospitalization needed to treat myoclonus, hypertension, and other symptoms.

Therapeutic Plasma Levels

Mood stabilizers

- Lithium: 1.0 – 1.5 mEq/L (acute mania)
  0.6 – 1.2 mEq/L (maintenance)
- Carbamazepine: 4 – 12 μg/mL
- Valproic acid: 50 – 100 μg/mL

NOTE: Lithium blood level should be drawn in the morning about 12 hours after last oral dose and before taking first morning dose.

DRUGS

Drug-Herbal Interactions

Antidepressants should not be used concurrently with: St. John's wort or SAMe (serotonin syndrome and/or altered antidepressant metabolism).

Benzodiazepines/sedative/hypnotics should not be used concurrently with chamomile, skullcap, valerian, or kava kava. St. John's wort may reduce the effectiveness of benzodiazepines metabolized by CYP P450 3A4.

Conventional antipsychotics (haloperidol, chlorpromazine) that are sedating should not be used in conjunction with chamomile, skullcap, valerian, or kava kava. Carbamazepine, clozapine, and olanzapine should not be used concurrently with St. John's wort (altered drug metabolism/effectiveness).

ALERT: Ask all clients specifically what, if any, herbal or OTC medications they are using to treat symptoms.

Antiparkinsonian Agents

Anticholinergics used to treat drug-induced parkinsonism, Parkinson's disease, and EPS. These include benztropine, biperiden, trihexyphenidyl, and others, including amantadine (dopaminergic) and diphenhydramine (antihistaminic) (see Psychotropic Drugs at www.fadavis.com/psychnotes). Anticholinergic side effects include blurred vision, dry mouth, constipation, sedation, urinary retention, and tachycardia. Use cautiously in the elderly and cardiac arrhythmias.

Note: Refer to the Physicians Desk Reference or Product Insert for complete drug and prescribing information (dosages, warnings, indications, adverse effects, interactions, etc.) needed to make appropriate choices in the treatment of clients. Although every effort has been made to provide key information about medications and classes of drugs, such information is not all inclusive and cannot be a reference of this nature. Professional judgment, training, supervision, relevant references, and current drug information are critical to the appropriate selection, evaluation, monitoring, and management of clients and their medications.

Common Psychotropic Medications (Alphabetical Listing)

Generic Name	Trade Name	Adult Dose Range	Geriatric Dose Considerations	Classification
Alprazolam	Xanax Xanax XR Apo-Alpraz	0.75–4 mg/d (anxiety); *panic:* not to exceed 10 mg/d; XR: usual range, 3–6 mg/d	↓ Dose required; begin 0.5–0.75 mg/d	Antianxiety agent
Amitriptyline	Elavil Apo-Amitriptyline Levate Novotriptyn	50–300 mg/d	Use caution: orthostatic hypotension, sedation, confusion (falls); CV disease; titrate slowly	Antidepressant
Aripiprazole	Abilify	10–15 mg/d (up to 30 mg/d)	Orthostatic hypotension; caution with CV disease/dementia	Antipsychotic
Benztropine	Cogentin Apo-Benztropine	Parkinsonism: 0.5–6 mg/d; EPS: 1–4 mg qd/bid; IM (acute dystonia): 1–2 mg	Use cautiously; ↑ risk adverse reactions	Antiparkinson agent

(Continued on following page)

(Continued)

Generic Name	Trade Name	Adult Dose Range	Geriatric Dose Considerations	Classification
Bupropion	Wellbutrin	200–450 mg/d	Use cautiously	Antidepressant
Buspirone	BuSpar	15–60 mg/d	Contraindicated: severe renal/hepatic disease	Antianxiety agent
Carbamazepine	Tegretol Apo-Carbamazepine	400–1200 mg/d	Use cautiously CV/hepatic disease; BPH	Anticonvulsant
Chlorpromazine	Thorazine Apo-Chlorpromazine	40–800 mg/d	Caution: sedating	Antipsychotic
Clomipramine	Anafranil Apo-Clomipramine	25–250 mg/d	Use with caution; CV disease; BPH	Antidepressant
Clonazepam	Klonopin Rivotril Syn-Clonazepam	1.5–6 mg/d (up to 20 mg/d [seizures])	Caution: drowsiness; contraindicated: liver disease	Antianxiety agent
Clozapine	Clozaril	300–900 mg/d	Use cautiously CV/hepatic/renal disease; sedating	Antipsychotic

Generic Name	Trade Name	Adult Dose Range	Geriatric Dose Considerations	Classification
Citalopram	Celexa	20–60 mg/d	Lower doses; hepatic/renal impairment	Antidepressant
Desipramine	Norpramin	25–300 mg/d	Reduce dosage; CV disease, BPH	Antidepressant
Diazepam	Valium Apo-Diazepam Vivol	4–40 mg/d	Dosage reduction required; hepatic/renal	Antianxiety agent
Divalproex sodium	Depakote Epival	500–1500 mg/d; titrate to clinical effect/plasma levels	Caution with renal/liver impairment, organic brain disease	Anticonvulsant
Doxepin	Sinequan Triadapin	25–300 mg/d	Dose reduction/CV disease, BPH, sedating	Antidepressant
Duloxetine	Cymbalta	40–60 mg/d	Use with caution; increase slowly	Antidepressant
Escitalopram	Lexapro	10–20 mg/d	↓ Dose; hepatic/renal impairment	Antidepressant

(Continued on following page)

(Continued)

Generic Name	Trade Name	Adult Dose Range	Geriatric Dose Considerations	Classification
Fluoxetine	Prozac Prozac Weekly Sarafem	20 mg/d (not to exceed 80 mg)	↓ dose (not to exceed 60 mg); hepatic/renal impairment; multiple medications (long T½)	Antidepressant
Fluvoxamine	Luvox	50–300 mg/d	Reduce dose, titrate slowly; Caution: impaired hepatic disease	Antidepressant
Fluphenazine	Prolixin Prolixin Decanoate *Modecate*	1–40 mg/d	Use lower doses; BPH, respiratory disease; contraindicated: severe liver/CV disease	Antipsychotic
Flurazepam	Dalmane *Apo-Flurazepam*	15–30 mg hs	Initial dose ↓; hepatic disease	Sedative/hypnotic
Gabapentin	Neurontin	900–1800 mg/d	Use cautiously	Anticonvulsant
Haloperidol	Haldol *Apo-Haloperidol Peridol*	1–100 mg/d	Dosage reduction required; *caution:* CV/diabetes, BPH	Antipsychotic

Generic Name	Trade Name	Adult Dose Range	Geriatric Dose Considerations	Classification
Hydroxyzine	Atarax; Vistaril Apo-Hydroxyzine	100–400 mg/d	Dosage reduction; severe hepatic disease	Antianxiety; sedative/ hypnotic
Imipramine	Tofranil Apo-Imipramine	30–300 mg/d	Use cautiously; CV disease/BPH	Antidepressant
Lamotrigine	Lamictal	75–250 mg/d	Impaired renal/CV/ hepatic disease	Anticonvulsant
Lithium	Eskalith Lithobid Carbolith Duralith	Acute mania: 1800–2400 mg/d; maintenance: 300–1200 mg/d	Initial dose reduction recommended; caution CV/renal/thyroid disease, diabetes mellitus	Antimanic
Lorazepam	Ativan Apo-Lorazepam	2–6 mg/d (up to 10 mg/d)	Dosage reduction; hepatic/renal/pul-monary	Antianxiety, sedative/ hypnotic
Loxapine	Loxitane	20–250 mg/d	Hypotension, sedation, CV events; ↓ dose	Antipsychotic
Mirtazapine	Remeron	15–45 mg/d	Lower dose; use cautiously hepatic/renal	Antidepressant

(Continued on following page)

(Continued)

Generic Name	Trade Name	Adult Dose Range	Geriatric Dose Considerations	Classification
Molindone	Moban	15–225 mg/d	Initial ↓ dose; diabetes, BPH, resp. disease	Antipsychotic
MAOIs: Phenelzine Tranylcypromine	Nardil Parnate	45–90 mg/d 30–60 mg/d	Use cautiously, titrate slowly	Antidepressant
Isocarboxazid	Marplan	20–60 mg/d		
Nadolol	Corgard; Syn-Nadolol	40 mg/d (up to 240 mg)	Initial dose reduction recommended	Antianginal; beta-blocker
Nefazodone	Serzone*	200–600 mg/d	Initiate lower dose HEPATIC FAILURE: HEPATIC TOXICITY	Antidepressant
Nortriptyline	Pamelor Aventyl	75–150 mg/d	↓ Dose: caution BPH, CV disease	Antidepressant
Olanzapine	Zyprexa Zyprexa Zydis	5–20 mg/d	Reduce dosage; CV, CVA, BPH, hepatic	Antipsychotic
Oxazepam	Serax Apo-Oxazepam	30–120 mg/d	↓ Dose: hepatic, severe COPD	Antianxiety

*Withdrawn from North American market (generic still available)

DRUGS

Generic Name	Trade Name	Adult Dose Range	Geriatric Dose Considerations	Classification
Paroxetine (do not use ≤ 18 y)	Paxil Paxil CR	10–60 mg/d; CR: 12.5–75 mg/d	← Dose; hepatic, renal impairment	Antidepressant/ antianxiety
Phenobarbital	Luminal Ancalixir	30–320 mg/d	Use cautiously: ↓ dose; hepatic/ renal disease	Sedative/ hypnotic
Pimozide	Orap	2–10 mg/d	Moderately sedating, Parkinson's, arrhythmias, QT prolongation, hypotension	Antipsychotic
Propranolol	Inderal Apo-Propranolol	80–120 mg/d (up to 320 mg/d) (tremors); akathisia: 30–120 mg/d	← Dose (elderly have increased sensitivity to beta-blockers); renal, hepatic, pulmonary disease, diabetes	Antianginal; beta-blocker
Quetiapine	Seroquel	150–800 mg/d	Cautiously in Alzheimer's, ≥65 y; CV/hepatic disease	Antipsychotic

(Continued on following page)

Generic Name	Trade Name	Adult Dose Range	Geriatric Dose Considerations	Classification
Risperidone	Risperdal	4–12 mg/d (over 6 mg ↑ risk of EPS; ≥10 mg EPS = haloperidol)	May ↑ stroke in elderly with dementia; caution: renal/hepatic disease/CV disease	Antipsychotic
Sertraline	Zoloft	50–200 mg/d	*Caution:* hepatic/renal impairment	Antidepressant
Thioridazine	Mellaril Apo-Thioridazine	150–800 mg/d	Use cautiously, CV disease, BPH	Antipsychotic
Topiramate	Topamax	50–400 mg/d (maximum dose: 1600 mg/d)	Adjust dose ↓ for renal/hepatic impairment	Anticonvulsant
Trazodone	Desyrel	150–400 mg/d (hospitalized up to 600 mg/d)	Reduced dose initially; titrate slowly; CV, hepatic, renal disease	Antidepressant/sedative

(Continued)

Generic Name	Trade Name	Adult Dose Range	Geriatric Dose Considerations	Classification
Venlafaxine	Effexor	75–225 mg/d; do not exceed 375 mg/d	Use cautiously with CV disease (hypertension).; reduce dose in renal/ hepatic impairment	Antidepressant
Ziprasidone	Geodon	40–160 mg/d (IM: 10–20 mg prn agitation (up to 40 mg/d)	↓ Dose in elderly; contraindicated: QT prolongation, CV disease & drugs; ≥65; Alzheimer's dementia	Antipsychotic
Zaleplon	Sonata	5–20 mg hs	Lower dose: age ≥ 65 or weigh ≤ 50 kg/hepatic im-pairment/con-current cimetidine	Sedative/ hypnotic
Zolpidem	Ambien	5–10 mg hs	Initial ↓ dose; hepatic disease	Sedative/ hypnotic

Crisis/Suicide/Abuse

Terrorism/Disasters

Terrorism/Disasters   (See Posttraumatic Stress Disorder, Stages of Death and Dying, and Complicated versus Uncomplicated Grief in the *Disorders Tab*; see also Suicide Assessment below)

Crisis Intervention

Phases

I. Assessment – What caused the crisis, and what are the individual's responses to it?

II. Planning intervention – Explore individual's strengths, weaknesses, support systems, and coping skills in dealing with the crisis.

III. Intervention – Establish relationship, help understand event and explore feelings, and explore alternative coping strategies.

IV. Evaluation/reaffirmation – Evaluate outcomes/plan for future/evaluate need for follow-up. (Aguilera 1998)

Prevention/Management of Assaultive Behaviors

Assessment of signs of anger is very important in prevention and in intervening *before anger escalates to assault/violence.*

Early Signs of Anger

- *Muscular tension*: clenched fist
- *Face*: furled brow, glaring eyes, tense mouth, clenched teeth, flushed face
- *Voice*: raised or lowered

If anger is not identified and recognized at **the preassaultive tension state,** this can progress to aggressive behavior.

Anger Management Techniques

- Remain calm
- Help client recognize anger
- Find an outlet: verbal (talking) or physical (exercise)
- Help client accept angry feelings; *not acceptable to act on them*
- Do not touch an angry client
- Medication may be needed

Signs of Anger Escalation

- Verbal/physical threats
- Pacing/appears agitated
- Throwing objects
- Appears suspicious/disproportionate anger
- Acts of violence/hitting

Anger Management Techniques
- Speak in short command sentences: *Joe, calm down.*
- Never allow yourself to be cornered with an angry client; *always have an escape route* (open door behind you)
- *Request assistance of other staff*
- Medication may be needed; *offer voluntarily first*
- Restraints and/or seclusion may be needed *(see Use of Restraints in Basics tab; also client restraint and management figures below)*
- Continue to *assess/reassess* (ongoing)
- When stabilized, *help client identify early signs/triggers of anger and alternatives* to prevent future anger/escalation

Walking client to the seclusion room (From Townsend MC. Psychiatric Mental Health Nursing: Concepts of Care, ed 3. Philadelphia: FA Davis, 2000, p. 219, with permission.)

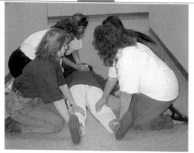

Restraint of client in a supine position by staff, controlling head to prevent biting. (From Townsend MC. Psychiatric Mental Health Nursing: Concepts of Care, ed 3. Philadelphia: FA Davis, 2000, p. 219, with permission.)

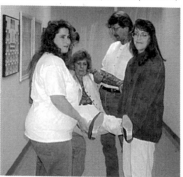

Transporting client to the seclusion room. (Townsend MC. Psychiatric Mental Health Nursing: Concepts of Care, ed 3. Philadelphia: FA Davis, 2000, p. 219, with permission.)

Suicide

Risk Factors Include:

- Mood disorders such as depression and bipolar disorder
- Substance abuse (dual diagnosis)
- Previous suicide attempt
- Loss – marital partner, partner, close relationship, job, health
- Expressed hopelessness or helplessness (does not see a future)
- Impulsivity/aggressiveness
- Family suicides, significant other or friend/peer suicide
- Isolation (lives alone/few friends, support relationships)
- Stressful life event
- Previous or current abuse (emotional/physical/sexual)
- Sexual identity crisis/conflict
- Available lethal method, such as a gun
- Legal issues/incarceration (USPHS, HHS 1999)

Suicide Assessment

- *Hopelessness* – A key element. Client is unable to see a future or self in that future.
- *Speaks of suicide (suicidal ideation)* – Important to ask client if he/she has thoughts of suicide and if so, should be considered suicidal.
- *Plan* – Client is able to provide an exact method for ending life. Must take seriously and consider immediacy of act.
- *Giving away possessions* – Any actions such as giving away possessions, putting affairs in order (recent will), connecting anew with old friends/family members.
- *Auditory hallucinations* – Commanding client to kill self.
- *Lack of support network* – Isolation, few friends or withdrawing from friends/support network.
- *Alcohol/other substance abuse* – Drinking alone.
- *Previous suicide attempt or family history of suicide.*
- *Precipitating event* – Death of a loved one; loss of a job, especially long-term job; holidays; tragedy; disaster.
- *Media* – Suicide of a famous personality or local teenager. (Rakel 2000)

CLINICAL PEARL – Do not confuse self-injurious behavior (cutting) with suicide attempts, although those who repeatedly cut themselves to relieve emotional pain could also attempt suicide. "Cutters" may want to stop cutting self but find stopping difficult, as this has become a *pattern of stress reduction*.

Groups at Risk for Suicide

- *Elderly* – especially those who are isolated, widowed; multiple losses, including friends/peers.
- *Males* – especially widowed and without close friends; sole emotional support came from marriage partner who is now deceased.
- *Adolescents and young adults*.
- *Serious/terminal illness* – not all terminally ill clients will be suicidal, but should be considered in those who become depressed or hopeless.
- *Mood disorders* – depression and especially bipolar. Always observe and assess those receiving treatment for depression, as suicide attempt may take place with improvement of depressive symptoms (client has the energy to commit suicide).
- *Schizophrenia* – newly diagnosed schizophrenics and those with command hallucinations.
- *Substance abusers* – especially with a mental disorder.
- *Stress and loss* – stressful situations and loss can trigger a suicide attempt, especially multiple stressors and losses, or a significant loss.

Suicide Interventions

- Effective assessment and knowledge of risk factors
- Observation and safe environment (no "sharps")
- Psychopharmacology, especially the SSRIs (children ≤18 y on SSRIs need to be closely monitored)
- Identification of triggers; educating client as to triggers to seek help early on

- Substance abuse treatment; treatment of pain disorders
- Psychotherapy/CBT/ECT
- Treatment of medical disorders (thyroid/cancer)
- Increased activity if able
- Support network/family involvement
- Involvement in outside activities/avoid isolation – join outside groups, bereavement groups, organizations, care for a pet
- Client and family education

Elder Suicide (See Geriatric Tab)

Victims of Abuse

Cycle of Battering

Phase I. Tension Building – Anger with little provocation; minor battering and excuses. Tension mounts and victim tries to placate. (Victim assumes guilt; *I deserve to be abused*.)

Phase II. Acute Battering – Most violent, up to 24 hours. Beating may be severe and victim may provoke to get it over. Minimized by abuser. Help sought by victim if life threatening or fear for children.

Phase III. Calm, Loving, Respite – Batterer is loving, kind, contrite. Fear of victim leaving. Lesson taught and now batterer believes victim "understands"

- Victim believes batterer can change and batterer uses guilt. Victim believes this (calm/loving in phase III) *is what batterer is really like*. Victim hopes the previous phases will not repeat themselves.
- Victim stays because of fear for life (batterer threatens more and self-esteem lowers); society values marriage, divorce is viewed negatively, financial dependence.

Starts all over again – dangerous, and victim often killed.

(Walker 1979)

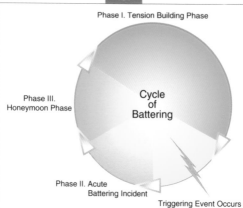

Cycle of battering. (From Townsend MC: Psychiatric Mental Health Nursing: Concepts of Care, ed 4. FA Davis, Philadelphia, 2003, p 776, with permission.)

Be aware that victims (of batterers) can be wives, husbands, intimate partners (female/female, male/male, male/female), and pregnant women.

Safety Plan (to Escape Abuser)

- Doors, windows, elevators – *rehearse exit plan.*
- *Have a place to go* – friends, relatives, motel – where you will be and feel safe.
- *Survival kit* – pack and *include money* (cab); change of clothes; identifying info (passports, birth certificate); legal documents, including protection orders; address books; jewelry; important papers.
- Start an *individual checking/savings account.*

- **Always have a safe exit** – do not argue in areas with no exit.
- Legal rights/domestic hotlines – know how to contact abuse/legal/domestic hotlines (see Website).
- Review safety plan consistently (monthly) (Reno 2004).

Signs of Child Abuse (Physical/Sexual)

Physical Abuse	Sexual Abuse
■ Pattern of bruises/welts	■ Signs of genital irritation, such as itching
■ Burns (e.g., from cigarettes, scalds)	■ Parent not providing
■ Lesions resembling bites or fingernail marks	■ Bruised or bleeding genitalia
■ Unexplained fractures or dislocations, especially in child younger than 3 yr	■ Enlarged vaginal or rectal orifice
■ Areas of baldness from hair pulling	■ Stains and/or blood on underwear
■ Injuries in various stages of healing	■ Unusual sexual behavior
■ Other injuries or untreated illness, unrelated to present injury	
■ X-rays revealing old fractures	

Signs Common to Both

- ■ Exaggeration or absence of emotional response from parent regarding child's injury
- ■ Parent not providing child with comfort
- ■ Toddler or preschooler not protesting parent's leaving
- ■ Child showing preference for health-care worker over parent
- ■ Signs of "failure to thrive" syndrome
- ■ Details of injury changing from person to person
- ■ History inconsistent with developmental stages
- ■ Parent blaming child or sibling for injury
- ■ Parental anger toward child for injury
- ■ Parental hostility toward health-care workers

Sources: Adapted from Myers RNotes 2003, page 38, with permission; Holloway BW: Nurse's Fast Facts: The Only Book You Need for Clinicals! Ed 3, FA Davis, Philadelphia, 2001; Miller JC, Stein AM: NSNA NCLEX-RN Review, ed 4, Delmar, New York, 2000, pp 486–487.

Child Abuser Characteristics
Characteristics associated with those who may be child abusers:

- Those in a stressful situation, such as unemployed
- Poor coping strategies; may be suspicious or lose temper easily
- Isolated, few support systems, or none
- Does not understand needs of children, basic care, or child development
- Expects child perfection and child behavior blown out of proportion (Murray and Zentner 1997)

Incest

Often a father-daughter relationship (biological/stepfather), but can be father-son as well as mother-son.

- Child is made to feel special ("It is our special secret"); gifts given
- Favoritism (becomes intimate friend/sex partner replacing mother/other parent)
- Serious boundary violations and no safe place for child (child's bedroom usually used)
- May be threats if child tells about the sexual activities. (Christianson and Blake 1990)

Signs of Incest:
- Low self esteem, sexual acting out, mood changes, sudden poor performance in school
- Parent spends inordinate amount of time with child, especially in room or late at night; very attentive to child
- Child is apprehensive (fearing sexual act/retaliation)
- Alcohol and drugs may be used (Christianson and Blake 1990)

ALERT: All child abuse (physical/sexual/emotional) or child neglect must be reported

Elder Abuse (See *Geriatric Tab*)

Other Kinds of Abuse

■ **Emotional Neglect** – Parental/caretaker behaviors include:
  ◆ ignoring child
  ◆ ignoring needs (social, educational, developmental)
  ◆ rebuffing child's attempts at establishing interactions that are meaningful
  ◆ little to no positive reinforcement (KCAPC 1992)

■ **Emotional Injury** – results in serious impairment in child's functioning on all levels:
  ◆ treatment of child is harsh, with cruel and negative comments, belittling child
  ◆ child may behave immaturely, with inappropriate behaviors for age
  ◆ demonstrates anxiety, fearfulness, sleep disturbances
  ◆ inappropriate affect, self-destructive behaviors
  ◆ may isolate, steal, cheat, as indication of emotional injury (KCAPC 1992)

■ **Male Sexual Abuse** – Males are also sexually abused by mothers, fathers, uncles, pedophiles, and others in authority (coach, teacher, minister, priest)
  ◆ suffer from depression, shame, blame, guilt, and other effects of child sexual abuse
  ◆ issues related to masculinity, isolation, and struggles with seeking or receiving help

Geriatric/Elderly

Decreased aortic elasticity	Produces increased diastolic blood pressure
Loss of subcutaneous tissue	Decreased insulation can put elderly at risk for hypothermia
Decreased skin vascularity	Altered thermoregulation response can put elderly at risk for heatstroke
Decreased skin thickness	Elderly clients are more prone to skin breakdown

Age-Related Changes and Their Implications

◆ Assess for altered mental states.
  - **Dementia:** Cognitive deficits (memory, reasoning, judgment, etc.)
  - **Delirium:** Confusion/excitement marked by disorientation to time and place, usually accompanied by illusions and/or hallucinations
  - **Depression:** Diminished interest or pleasure in most/all activities

Geriatric Assessment

Key Points

◆ Be mindful that the elderly client may be hard of hearing, but do not assume that all elderly are hard of hearing.

◆ Approach and speak to elderly clients as you would to any other adult client. It is insulting to speak to the elderly client as if he/she were a child.

◆ Eye contact helps instill confidence and, in the presence of impaired hearing, will help the client to better understand you.

◆ Be aware that both decreased tactile sensation and ROM are normal changes with aging. Care should be taken to avoid unnecessary discomfort or even injury during a physical exam/assessment.

◆ Be aware of generational differences, especially gender differences (i.e., modesty for women, independence for men).

Calcification of thoracic wall	Obscures heart and lung sounds and displaces apical pulse
Loss of nerve fibers/neurons	The elderly client needs extra time to learn and comprehend and to perform certain tasks
Decreased nerve conduction	Response to pain is altered
Reduced tactile sensation	Puts client at risk for accidental self-injury

From Myers RNotes 2003, p. 40, with permission

Disorders of Late Life

- **Dementia** – Dementia of the Alzheimer's type (AD), dementia with Lewy bodies, vascular and other dementias, delirium, and amnestic disorder. (*See Delirium, Dementia, and Amnestic Disorders in the Disorders Tab.*)
- **Geriatric depression** – Depression in old age is often assumed to be normal; however, depression at any age is not normal and needs to be diagnosed and treated. Factors can include
  - ◆ physical and cognitive decline
  - ◆ loss of function/self-sufficiency
  - ◆ loss of marriage partner, friends (narrowing support group), isolation
  - ◆ The elderly may have many somatic complaints (head hurts, stomach upsets) that mask the depression. (Chenitz 1991) (*See Geriatric Depression Scale in Assessment Tab*)
- **Pseudodementia** – Cognitive difficulty that is *actually caused by depression but may be mistaken for dementia.*
  - ◆ Need to consider and rule out dementia (MMSE) and actually differentiate from depression (GDS)
  - ◆ Can be depressed with cognitive deficits as well
- **Late-onset schizophrenia** – Presents later in life, after age 60.
  - ◆ Psychotic episodes (delusions or hallucinations) may be overlooked (schizophrenia is considered to be a young-adult disease)
  - ◆ Organic brain disease should be considered as part of the differential diagnosis

Characteristics of Late-Onset Schizophrenia

- *Delusions of persecution* are common, *hallucinations* prominent; also *"partition" delusion* (people/objects pass through barriers and enter home) common; rare in early onset
- *Sensory deficits* – often auditory/visual impairments
- May have been *previously paranoid, reclusive*, yet functioned otherwise
- *Lives alone/isolated/unmarried*
- *Negative symptoms/thought disorder* rare
- **More common in women** (early onset; equally common) (Lubman & Castle 2002)

Psychotropic Drugs – Geriatric Considerations
(See Drug Tab for alphabetical listing of Common Psychotropic Medications and also Medications and the Elderly.)

Pharmacokinetics in the Elderly

Pharmacokinetics is the way that a drug is absorbed, distributed and used, metabolized, and excreted by the body. Age-related physiological changes affect body systems, altering pharmacokinetics and increasing or altering a drug's effect.

	Physiological Change	Effect on Pharmacokinetics
Absorption	■ Decreased intestinal motility ■ Diminished blood flow to the gut	■ Delayed peak effect ■ Delayed signs/ symptoms of toxic effects
Distribution	■ Decreased body water ■ Increased percentage of body fat ■ Decreased amount of plasma proteins ■ Decreased lean body mass	■ Increased serum concentration of water-soluble drugs ■ Increased half-life of fat-soluble drugs ■ Increased amount of active drug ■ Increased drug concentration

	Physiological Change	Effect on Pharmacokinetics
Metabolism	■ Decreased blood flow to liver	■ Decreased rate of drug clearance by liver
	■ Diminished liver function	■ Increased accumulation of some drugs
Excretion	■ Diminished kidney function ■ Decreased creatinine clearance	■ Increased accumulation of drugs excreted by kidney

From Myers LPN Notes 2004, p. 76, with permission

Common Medications for the Elderly – Potential Problems

Cardiovascular and Antihypertensive

Digoxin (e.g., Lanoxin, Lanoxicaps)

■ Digitalis toxicity occurs more frequently in the elderly. Cardiac arrhythmias and conduction disturbances are the first signs of toxicity more often than nausea, anorexia, and visual disturbances.
■ The risk for digoxin toxicity is greater when given with drugs such as verapamil, amiodarone, or quinidine.
■ **Monitor carefully when digoxin is given with diuretics.** They can potentiate digitalis toxicity.

Thiazides (e.g., HydroDIURIL, Zaroxolyn, Exna)

■ Thiazides cause greater potassium loss in elderly patients. Potassium supplementation is often necessary.
■ Thiazides can cause low serum sodium (hyponatremia), which can manifest as delirium.

(Continued on following page)

Beta-Blockers (e.g., Brevibloc, Inderal, Blocadren)

- Can worsen heart failure, asthma, and emphysema.
- Lipid-soluble beta-blockers (propranolol and metoprolol) cross the blood-brain barrier more easily than water-soluble beta-blockers (atenolol, nadolol) and have a greater potential to produce CNS adverse reactions such as vivid dreams, fatigue, and depression.

Calcium Channel Blockers (e.g., Adalat, Calan, Cardizem)

- Can worsen heart failure.

H2 Histamine Antagonists (e.g., Zantac, Tagamet, Pepcid)

- Cimetidine interferes with the metabolism of phenytoin, carbamazepine, theophylline, warfarin, and quinidine and increases the half-life. Ranitidine has a similar but lesser effect.
- Cimetidine has been associated with confusion, psychosis, and hallucinations, most commonly in elderly and/or severely ill patients. These CNS effects resolve within a few days after discontinuation of the drug.

Nonsteroidal Anti-inflammatory Drugs (NSAIDs) (e.g., ibuprofen [Advil, Motrin])

- Gastric ulceration and bleeding are common in patients taking NSAIDs on a chronic basis.
- There are often no warning signs, such as abdominal pain or nausea, of NSAID-induced gastric bleeding.
- The first symptom of GI toxicity in many elderly is upper GI hemorrhage.
- Acute tubular necrosis and renal failure also occur with use of NSAIDs.

Psychotropic Drugs

Neuroleptics/Antipsychotics (see Drug tab)

- Neuroleptics lower blood pressure and may worsen orthostatic hypotension.
- May cause increased confusion, dry mouth, constipation, and/or urinary retention.
- Tardive dyskinesia can develop in the elderly even with short-term, low-dose use.

(Continued)

Tricyclic Antidepressants (see *Drug tab*)

- Can aggravate and contraindicated in glaucoma.
- Can cause urinary retention.
- Amitriptyline can cause severe hypotension in the elderly.

Benzodiazepines (see *Drug tab*)

- Can be addictive.
- Can accumulate in the elderly and cause daytime **sleepiness, confusion, and an increased risk of falls**.
- Shorter acting benzodiazepines have less tendency to accumulate.
- Daily long-term use and long-acting products should be avoided whenever possible.

Modified from Myers LPN Notes 2004, p. 79, with permission

Elder Abuse

There are many types of elder abuse, which include:
- *elder neglect* (lack of care by omission or commission)
- *psychological or emotional abuse* (verbal assaults, insults, threats)
- *physical* (physical injury, pain, drugs, restraints)
- *sexual abuse* (nonconsensual sex: rape, sodomy)
- *financial abuse* (misuse of resources: social security, property)
- *self neglect* (elder cannot provide appropriate self care)

Elder Abuse – Physical Signs

- Hematomas, welts, bites, burns, bruises, and pressure sores
- Fractures (various stages of healing), contractures
- Rashes, fecal impaction
- Weight loss, dehydration, substandard personal hygiene
- Broken dentures, hearing aids, other devices; poor oral hygiene; traumatic alopecia; subconjunctival hemorrhage

Elder Abuse – Behavioral Signs

Caregiver

- Caregiver insistence on being present during entire appointment
- Answers for client

- Expresses indifference or anger, not offering assistance
- Caregiver does not visit hospitalized client

Elder
- Hesitation to be open, appearing fearful, poor eye contact, ashamed, baby talk
- Paranoia, anxiety, anger, low self esteem
- *Physical signs:* contractures, inconsistent medication regimen (subtherapeutic levels), malnutrition, poor hygiene, dehydration
- *Financial:* signed over POA (unwillingly), possessions gone, lack of money

Elder Abuse – Medical and Psychiatric History
- Mental health/psychiatric interview
- Assess for depression, anxiety, alcohol (substance) abuse, insomnia
- Functional independence/dependence
- Cognitive impairment

(Stiles et al. 2002)

ALERT: All elder abuse must be reported.

Elder Suicide

Warning Signs
- Failed suicide attempt
- *Indirect clues* – stockpiling medications; purchasing a gun; putting affairs in order; making/changing a will; donating body to science; giving possessions/money away; relationship, social downturns; recent appointment with a physician
- *Situational clues* – recent move, death of spouse or friend or child
- *Symptoms* – depression, insomnia, agitation, others

Elder Profile for Potential Suicide
- Male gender
- White
- Divorced or widowed
- Lives alone, isolated, moved recently
- Unemployed, retired

- Poor health, pain, multiple illnesses, terminal
- Depressed, substance abuser, hopeless
- Family history of suicide, depression, substance abuse. Harsh parenting, early trauma in childhood
- Wish to end hopeless, intolerable situation
- *Lethal means*: guns, stockpiled sedatives/hypnotics
- Previous attempt
- Not inclined to reach out; often somatic complaints

Suspected Elder Suicidality
Ask direct questions:
- Are you so down you see no point in going on? (If answer is yes, explore further: *Tell me more*)
- Have you (ever) thought of killing yourself? (*When; what stopped you?*)
- How often do you have these thoughts?
- How would you kill yourself? (Lethality plan)

(Holkup 2002)

Gather information – keep communication open in a nonjudgmental way; do not minimize or offer advice in this situation.

Tools

Note: The following additional resources can be found on the PsychNotes Website:

■ Psychiatric Assessment Rating Scale Information
■ NANDA Nursing Diagnoses: Taxonomy II
■ Psychiatric Resources/Organizations/Websites/Hotlines

Go to: **http://www.fadavis.com/psychnotes/**

Community Resources/Phone Numbers

Name/Program	Phone Number

Sexual and Physical Abuse

Substance Abuse

Communicable Disease (AIDs/Hepatitis)

Homeless Shelters

Child/Adolescent Hotlines

Suicide Hotlines

Hospitals (Medical/Psychiatric)

Other

Abbreviations

AD Dementia of Alzheimer's type

ADHD Attention deficit hyperactivity disorder

AE Adverse event

AIMS Abnormal Involuntary Movement Scale

BAI Beck Anxiety Inventory

BDI Beck Depression Inventory

BP Blood pressure

BPD Borderline personality disorder

BPH Benign prostatic hypertrophy

CBC Complete blood count

CBT Cognitive behavioral therapy

CHF Congestive heart failure

CK Creatine kinase

CNS Central nervous system

COPD Chronic obstructive pulmonary disease

CT scan Computed tomography scan

CV Cardiovascular

DBT Dialectical behavioral therapy

d/c Discontinue

ECA Epidemiologic Catchment Area Survey

ECG Electrocardiogram

ECT Electroconvulsive therapy

EMDR Eye movement desensitization & reprocessing

EPS Extrapyramidal symptoms

FBS Fasting blood sugar

GABA Gamma-aminobutyric acid

GAD Generalized anxiety disorder

GDS Geriatric Depression Scale

Hx History

LFTs Liver function tests

IM Intramuscular

IV Intravenous

kg Kilogram

L Liter

MAOI Monoamine oxidase inhibitor

MCV Mean corpuscular volume

MDD Major depressive disorder

mEq Milliequivalent

μg Microgram

MH Mental health

mL Milliliter

MMSE Mini-Mental State Exam

MRI Magnetic resonance imaging

MSE Mental Status Exam

NAMI National Association for the Mentally Ill

NE Norepinephrine

NMS Neuroleptic malignant syndrome

OCD Obsessive-compulsive disorder

OCPD Obsessive-compulsive personality disorder

OTC Over the counter

PANSS Positive and Negative Syndrome Scale

(Continued on following page)

(Continued)	
PMDD Premenstrual dysphoric disorder	**T$^1/_2$** Drug's half life
PTSD Posttraumatic stress disorder	**TCA** Tricyclic antidepressant
	TFT Thyroid function test
SMAST Short Michigan Alcohol screening Test	**TIA** Transient ischemic attack
	TPR Temperature, pulse, respiration
SNRI Serotonin-norepinephrine reuptake inhibitor	**UA** Urinalysis
	UTI Urinary tract infection
SSRI Selective serotonin reuptake inhibitor	

Assessment Tools

See Assessment Tab for the following tools:

- Abnormal Involuntary Movement Scale (AIMS)
- CAGE Screening Quesionnaire
- DSM-IV Multiaxial Assessment Tool
- Geriatric Depression Scale (GDS)
- Global Assessment of Functioning (GAF) Scale
- Ethnocultural Assessment Tool
- Mental Status Assessment Tool
- Psychiatric History and Assessment Tool
- Short Michigan Alcohol Screening Test (SMAST)
- Substance History and Assessment

DSM-IV-TR Classification: Axes I and II Categories and Codes

DISORDERS USUALLY FIRST DIAGNOSED IN INFANCY, CHILDHOOD, OR ADOLESCENCE
  Mental Retardation
NOTE: *These are coded on Axis II.*
317 Mild Mental Retardation
318.0 Moderate Retardation
318.1 Severe Retardation

318.2 Profound Mental Retardation
319 Mental Retardation, Severity Unspecified
Learning Disorders
315.00 Reading Disorder
315.1 Mathematics Disorder
315.2 Disorder of Written Expression
315.9 Learning Disorder Not Otherwise Specified (NOS)
Motor Skills Disorder
315.4 Developmental Coordination Disorder
Communication Disorders
315.31 Expressive Language Disorder
315.32 Mixed Receptive-Expressive Language Disorder
315.39 Phonological Disorder
307.0 Stuttering
307.9 Communication Disorder NOS
Pervasive Developmental Disorders
299.00 Autistic Disorder
299.80 Rett's Disorder
299.10 Childhood Disintegrative Disorder
299.80 Asperger's Disorder
299.80 Pervasive Developmental Disorder NOS
Attention-Deficit and Disruptive Behavior Disorders
314.xx Attention-Deficit/Hyperactivity Disorder
314.01 Combined Type
314.00 Predominantly Inattentive Type
314.01 Predominantly Hyperactive-Impulsive Type
314.9 Attention-Deficit/Hyperactivity Disorder NOS
312.xx Conduct Disorder
.81 Childhood-Onset Type
.82 Adolescent-Onset Type
.89 Unspecified Onset
313.81 Oppositional Defiant Disorder
312.9 Disruptive Behavior Disorder NOS
Feeding and Eating Disorders of Infancy or Early Childhood
307.52 Pica
307.53 Rumination Disorder
307.59 Feeding Disorder of Infancy or Early Childhood

Tic Disorders
307.23 Tourette's Disorder
307.22 Chronic Motor or Vocal Tic Disorder
307.21 Transient Tic Disorder
307.20 Tic Disorder NOS

Elimination Disorders
—.— Encopresis
787.6 With Constipation and Overflow Incontinence
307.7 Without Constipation and Overflow Incontinence
307.6 Enuresis (Not Due to a General Medical Condition)

Other Disorders of Infancy, Childhood, or Adolescence
309.21 Separation Anxiety Disorder
313.23 Selective Mutism
313.89 Reactive Attachment Disorder of Infancy or Early Childhood
307.3 Stereotypic Movement Disorder
313.9 Disorder of Infancy, Childhood, or Adolescence NOS

DELIRIUM, DEMENTIA, AND AMNESTIC AND OTHER COGNITIVE DISORDERS

Delirium
293.0 Delirium Due to... (*Indicate the general medical condition*)
—.— Substance Intoxication Delirium (*refer to Substance-Related Disorders for substance-specific codes*)
—.— Substance Withdrawal Delirium (*refer to Substance-Related Disorders for substance-specific codes*)
—.— Delirium Due to Multiple Etiologies (*code each of the specific etiologies*)
780.09 Delirium NOS

Dementia
294.xx* Dementia of the Alzheimer's Type, With Early Onset
.10 Without Behavioral Disturbance
.11 With Behavioral Disturbance
294.xx* Dementia of the Alzheimer's Type, With Late Onset
.10 Without Behavioral Disturbance
.11 With Behavioral Disturbance

290.xx Vascular Dementia
   .40 Uncomplicated
   .41 With Delirium
   .42 With Delusions
   .43 With Depressed Mood
294.1x* Dementia Due to HIV Disease
294.1x* Dementia Due to Head Trauma
294.1x* Dementia Due to Parkinson's Disease
294.1x* Dementia Due to Huntington's Disease
294.1x* Dementia Due to Pick's Disease
294.1x* Dementia Due to Creutzfeldt-Jakob Disease
294.1x* Dementia Due to (*Indicate the general medical condition not listed above*)
—.— Substance-Induced Persisting Dementia (refer to Substance-Related Disorders for substance-specific codes)
—.— Dementia Due to Multiple Etiologies (code each of the specific etiologies)
294.8 Dementia NOS

Amnestic Disorders

294.0 Amnestic Disorder Due to (*Indicate the general medical condition*)
—.— Substance-Induced Persisting Amnestic Disorder (*refer to Substance-Related Disorders for substance-specific codes*)
294.8 Amnestic Disorder NOS

Other Cognitive Disorders

294.9 Cognitive Disorder NOS

MENTAL DISORDERS DUE TO A GENERAL MEDICAL CONDITION NOT ELSEWHERE CLASSIFIED
293.89 Catatonic Disorder Due to (*Indicate the general medical condition*)
310.1 Personality Change Due to (*Indicate the general medical condition*)
293.9 Mental Disorder NOS Due to (*Indicate the general medical condition*)

*Also add ICD-9-CM codes valid after October 1, 2000 on Axis III for these disorders.

SUBSTANCE-RELATED DISORDERS

Alcohol-Related Disorders

Alcohol Use Disorders
303.90 Alcohol Dependence
305.00 Alcohol Abuse
Alcohol-Induced Disorders
303.00 Alcohol Intoxication
291.81 Alcohol Withdrawal
291.0 Alcohol Intoxication Delirium
291.0 Alcohol Withdrawal Delirium
291.2 Alcohol-Induced Persisting Dementia
291.1 Alcohol-Induced Persisting Amnestic Disorder
291.x Alcohol-Induced Psychotic Disorder
   .5 With Delusions
   .3 With Hallucinations
291.89 Alcohol-Induced Mood Disorder
291.89 Alcohol-Induced Anxiety Disorder
291.89 Alcohol-Induced Sexual Dysfunction
291.89 Alcohol-Induced Sleep Disorder
291.9 Alcohol-Related Disorder NOS

Amphetamine (or Amphetamine-like)-Related Disorders

Amphetamine Use Disorders
304.40 Amphetamine Dependence
305.70 Amphetamine Abuse
Amphetamine-Induced Disorders
292.89 Amphetamine Intoxication
292.0 Amphetamine Withdrawal
292.81 Amphetamine Intoxication Delirium
292.xx Amphetamine-Induced Psychotic Disorder
   .11 With Delusions
   .12 With Hallucinations
292.84 Amphetamine-Induced Mood Disorder
292.89 Amphetamine-Induced Anxiety Disorder
292.89 Amphetamine-Induced Sexual Dysfunction
292.89 Amphetamine-Induced Sleep Disorder
292.9 Amphetamine-Related Disorder NOS

Caffeine-Related Disorders
Caffeine-Induced Disorders
305.90 Caffeine Intoxication
292.89 Caffeine-Induced Anxiety Disorder
292.89 Caffeine-Induced Sleep Disorder
292.9 Caffeine-Related Disorder NOS
 Cannabis-Related Disorders
Cannabis Use Disorders
304.30 Cannabis Dependence
305.20 Cannabis Abuse
Cannabis-Induced Disorders
292.89 Cannabis Intoxication
292.81 Cannabis Intoxication Delirium
292.xx Cannabis-Induced Psychotic Disorder
    .11 With Delusions
    .12 With Hallucinations
292.89 Cannabis-Induced Anxiety Disorder
292.9 Cannabis-Related Disorder NOS
Cocaine-Related Disorders
Cocaine Use Disorders
304.20 Cocaine Dependence
305.60 Cocaine Abuse
Cocaine-Induced Disorders
292.89 Cocaine Intoxication
292.0 Cocaine Withdrawal
292.81 Cocaine Intoxication Delirium
292.xx Cocaine-Induced Psychotic Disorder
    .11 With Delusions
    .12 With Hallucinations
292.84 Cocaine-Induced Mood Disorder
292.89 Cocaine-Induced Anxiety Disorder
292.89 Cocaine-Induced Sexual Dysfunction
292.89 Cocaine-Induced Sleep Disorder
292.9 Cocaine-Related Disorder NOS

Hallucinogen-Related Disorders
Hallucinogen Use Disorders
304.50 Hallucinogen Dependence
305.30 Hallucinogen Abuse
Hallucinogen-Induced Disorders
292.89 Hallucinogen Intoxication
292.89 Hallucinogen Persisting Perception Disorder (Flashbacks)
292.81 Hallucinogen Intoxication Delirium
292.xx Hallucinogen-Induced Psychotic Disorder
.11 With Delusions
.12 With Hallucinations
292.84 Hallucinogen-Induced Mood Disorder
292.89 Hallucinogen-Induced Anxiety Disorder
292.9 Hallucinogen-Related Disorder NOS
Inhalant-Related Disorders
Inhalant Use Disorders
304.60 Inhalant Dependence
305.90 Inhalant Abuse
Inhalant-Induced Disorders
292.89 Inhalant Intoxication
292.81 Inhalant Intoxication Delirium
292.82 Inhalant-Induced Persisting Dementia
292.xx Inhalant-Induced Psychotic Disorder
.11 With Delusions
.12 With Hallucinations
292.84 Inhalant-Induced Mood Disorder
292.89 Inhalant-Induced Anxiety Disorder
292.9 Inhalant-Related Disorder NOS
Nicotine-Related Disorders
Nicotine Use Disorders
305.1 Nicotine Dependence
Nicotine-Induced Disorders
292.0 Nicotine Withdrawal
292.9 Nicotine-Related Disorder NOS
Opioid-Related Disorders
Opioid Use Disorders
304.00 Opioid Dependence
305.50 Opioid Abuse

Opioid-Induced Disorders
292.89 Opioid Intoxication
292.0 Opioid Withdrawal
292.81 Opioid Intoxication Delirium
292.xx Opioid-Induced Psychotic Disorder
　.11 With Delusions
　.12 With Hallucinations
292.84 Opioid-Induced Mood Disorder
292.89 Opioid-Induced Sexual Dysfunction
292.89 Opioid-Induced Sleep Disorder
292.9 Opioid-Related Disorder NOS

Phencyclidine (or Phencyclidine-like)–Related Disorders
Phencyclidine Use Disorders
304.60 Phencyclidine Dependence
305.90 Phencyclidine Abuse
Phencyclidine-Induced Disorders
292.89 Phencyclidine Intoxication
292.81 Phencyclidine Intoxication Delirium
292.xx Phencyclidine-Induced Psychotic Disorder
　.11 With Delusions
　.12 With Hallucinations
292.84 Phencyclidine-Induced Mood Disorder
292.89 Phencyclidine-Induced Anxiety Disorder
292.9 Phencyclidine-Related Disorder NOS

Sedative-, Hypnotic-, or Anxiolytic-Related Disorders
Sedative, Hypnotic, or Anxiolytic Use Disorders
304.10 Sedative, Hypnotic, or Anxiolytic Dependence
305.40 Sedative, Hypnotic, or Anxiolytic Abuse
Sedative-, Hypnotic-, or Anxiolytic-Induced Disorders
292.89 Sedative, Hypnotic, or Anxiolytic Intoxication
292.0 Sedative, Hypnotic, or Anxiolytic Withdrawal
292.81 Sedative, Hypnotic, or Anxiolytic Intoxication Delirium
292.81 Sedative, Hypnotic, or Anxiolytic Withdrawal Delirium
292.82 Sedative-, Hypnotic-, or Anxiolytic-Induced Persisting Dementia
292.83 Sedative-, Hypnotic-, or Anxiolytic-Induced Persisting Amnestic Disorder

292.xx Sedative-, Hypnotic-, or Anxiolytic-Induced Psychotic
   Disorder
   .11 With Delusions
   .12 With Hallucinations
292.84 Sedative-, Hypnotic-, or Anxiolytic-Induced Mood
   Disorder
292.89 Sedative-, Hypnotic-, or Anxiolytic-Induced Anxiety
   Disorder
292.89 Sedative-, Hypnotic-, or Anxiolytic-Induced Sexual
   Dysfunction
292.89 Sedative-, Hypnotic-, or Anxiolytic-Induced Sleep Disorder
292.9 Sedative-, Hypnotic-, or Anxiolytic-Related Disorder NOS

Polysubstance-Related Disorder
304.80 Polysubstance Dependence

Other (or Unknown) Substance-Related Disorders
Other (or Unknown) Substance Use Disorders
304.90 Other (or Unknown) Substance Dependence
305.90 Other (or Unknown) Substance Abuse
Other (or Unknown) Substance-Induced Disorders
292.89 Other (or Unknown) Substance Intoxication
292.0 Other (or Unknown) Substance Withdrawal
292.81 Other (or Unknown) Substance-Induced Delirium
292.82 Other (or Unknown) Substance-Induced Persisting
   Dementia
292.83 Other (or Unknown) Substance-Induced Persisting
   Amnestic Disorder
292.xx Other (or Unknown) Substance-Induced Psychotic
   Disorder
   .11 With Delusions
   .12 With Hallucinations
292.84 Other (or Unknown) Substance-Induced Mood Disorder
292.89 Other (or Unknown) Substance-Induced Anxiety Disorder
292.89 Other (or Unknown) Substance-Induced Sexual
   Dysfunction
292.89 Other (or Unknown) Substance-Induced Sleep Disorder
292.9 Other (or Unknown) Substance-Related Disorder NOS

SCHIZOPHRENIA AND OTHER PSYCHOTIC DISORDERS
295.xx Schizophrenia
   .30 Paranoid type
   .10 Disorganized type
   .20 Catatonic type
   .90 Undifferentiated type
   .60 Residual type
295.40 Schizophreniform Disorder
295.70 Schizoaffective Disorder
297.1 Delusional Disorder
298.8 Brief Psychotic Disorder
297.3 Shared Psychotic Disorder
293.xx Psychotic Disorder Due to (*Indicate the general medical condition*)
   .81 With Delusions
   .82 With Hallucinations
—.— Substance-Induced Psychotic Disorder (*refer to Substance-Related Disorders for substance-specific codes*)
298.9 Psychotic Disorder NOS

MOOD DISORDERS
(Code current state of Major Depressive Disorder or Bipolar I Disorder in fifth digit: 0 = unspecified; 1 = mild; 2 = moderate; 3 = severe, without psychotic features; 4 = severe, with psychotic features; 5 = in partial remission; 6 = in full remission.)
Depressive Disorders
296.xx Major Depressive Disorder
   .2x Single Episode
   .3x Recurrent
300.4 Dysthymic Disorder
311 Depressive Disorder NOS
Bipolar Disorders
296.xx Bipolar I Disorder
   .0x Single Manic Episode
   .40 Most Recent Episode Hypomanic
   .4x Most Recent Episode Manic
   .6x Most Recent Episode Mixed

.5x Most Recent Episode Depressed
.7 Most Recent Episode Unspecified
296.89 Bipolar II Disorder (*Specify current or most recent episode: Hypomanic or Depressed*)
301.13 Cyclothymic Disorder
296.80 Bipolar Disorder NOS
293.83 Mood Disorder Due to (*Indicate the general medical condition*)
—.— Substance-Induced Mood Disorder (*refer to Substance-Related Disorders for substance-specific codes*)
296.90 Mood Disorder NOS

ANXIETY DISORDERS
300.01 Panic Disorder Without Agoraphobia
300.21 Panic Disorder With Agoraphobia
300.22 Agoraphobia Without History of Panic Disorder
300.29 Specific Phobia
300.23 Social Phobia
300.3 Obsessive-Compulsive Disorder
309.81 Posttraumatic Stress Disorder
308.3 Acute Stress Disorder
300.02 Generalized Anxiety Disorder
293.89 Anxiety Disorder Due to (*Indicate the general medical condition*)
—.— Substance-Induced Anxiety Disorder (*refer to Substance-Related Disorders for substance-specific codes*)
300.00 Anxiety Disorder NOS

SOMATOFORM DISORDERS
300.81 Somatization Disorder
300.82 Undifferentiated Somatoform Disorder
300.11 Conversion Disorder
307.xx Pain Disorder
  .80 Associated with Psychological Factors
  .89 Associated with Both Psychological Factors and a General Medical Condition
300.7 Hypochondriasis
300.7 Body Dysmorphic Disorder
300.82 Somatoform Disorder NOS

FACTITIOUS DISORDERS
300.xx Factitious Disorder
    .16 With Predominantly Psychological Signs and Symptoms
    .19 With Predominantly Physical Signs and Symptoms
    .19 With Combined Psychological and Physical Signs and
    Symptoms
300.19 Factitious Disorder NOS

DISSOCIATIVE DISORDERS
300.12 Dissociative Amnesia
300.13 Dissociative Fugue
300.14 Dissociative Identity Disorder
300.6 Depersonalization Disorder
300.15 Dissociative Disorder NOS

SEXUAL AND GENDER IDENTITY DISORDERS
Sexual Dysfunctions
Sexual Desire Disorders
302.71 Hypoactive Sexual Desire Disorder
302.79 Sexual Aversion Disorder
Sexual Arousal Disorders
302.72 Female Sexual Arousal Disorder
302.72 Male Erectile Disorder
Orgasmic Disorders
302.73 Female Orgasmic Disorder
302.74 Male Orgasmic Disorder
302.75 Premature Ejaculation
Sexual Pain Disorders
302.76 Dyspareunia (Not Due to a General Medical Condition)
306.51 Vaginismus (Not Due to a General Medical Condition)
Sexual Dysfunction Due to a General Medical Condition
625.8 Female Hypoactive Sexual Desire Disorder Due to (Indicate
the general medical condition)
608.89 Male Hypoactive Sexual Desire Disorder Due to (Indicate
the general medical condition)
607.84 Male Erectile Disorder Due to (Indicate the general
medical condition)
625.0 Female Dyspareunia Due to (Indicate the general medical
condition)

608.89 Male Dyspareunia Due to (Indicate the general medical condition)
625.8 Other Female Sexual Dysfunction Due to (Indicate the general medical condition)
608.89 Other Male Sexual Dysfunction Due to (Indicate the general medical condition)
—.— Substance-Induced Sexual Dysfunction (refer to Substance-Related Disorders for substance-specific codes)
302.70 Sexual Dysfunction NOS

Paraphilias
302.4 Exhibitionism
302.81 Fetishism
302.89 Frotteurism
302.2 Pedophilia
302.83 Sexual Masochism
302.84 Sexual Sadism
302.3 Transvestic Fetishism
302.82 Voyeurism
302.9 Paraphilia NOS

Gender Identity Disorders
302.xx Gender Identity Disorder
    .6 In Children
    .85 In Adolescents or Adults
302.6 Gender Identity Disorder NOS
302.9 Sexual Disorder NOS

EATING DISORDERS
307.1 Anorexia Nervosa
307.51 Bulimia Nervosa
307.50 Eating Disorder NOS

SLEEP DISORDERS
Primary Sleep Disorders
  Dyssomnias
307.42 Primary Insomnia
307.44 Primary Hypersomnia
347 Narcolepsy
780.59 Breathing-Related Sleep Disorder
307.45 Circadian Rhythm Sleep Disorder
307.47 Dyssomnia NOS

Parasomnias
307.47 Nightmare Disorder
307.46 Sleep Terror Disorder
307.46 Sleepwalking Disorder
307.47 Parasomnia NOS
Sleep Disorders Related to Another Mental Disorder
307.42 Insomnia Related to (Indicate the Axis I or Axis II disorder)
307.44 Hypersomnia Related to (Indicate the Axis I or Axis II disorder)
Other Sleep Disorders
780.xx Sleep Disorder Due to (Indicate the general medical condition)
    .52 Insomnia type
    .54 Hypersomnia type
    .59 Parasomnia type
    .59 Mixed type
Substance-Induced Sleep Disorder (refer to Substance-Related Disorders for substance-specific codes)

IMPULSE CONTROL DISORDERS NOT ELSEWHERE CLASSIFIED
312.34 Intermittent Explosive Disorder
312.32 Kleptomania
312.33 Pyromania
312.31 Pathological Gambling
312.39 Trichotillomania
312.30 Impulse Control Disorder NOS

ADJUSTMENT DISORDERS
309.xx Adjustment Disorder
    .0 With Depressed Mood
    .24 With Anxiety
    .28 With Mixed Anxiety and Depressed Mood
    .3 With Disturbance of Conduct
    .4 With Mixed Disturbance of Emotions and Conduct
    .9 Unspecified

PERSONALITY DISORDERS

NOTE: *These are coded on Axis II.*

301.0 Paranoid Personality Disorder
301.20 Schizoid Personality Disorder
301.22 Schizotypal Personality Disorder
301.7 Antisocial Personality Disorder
301.83 Borderline Personality Disorder
301.50 Histrionic Personality Disorder
301.81 Narcissistic Personality Disorder
301.82 Avoidant Personality Disorder
301.6 Dependent Personality Disorder
301.4 Obsessive-Compulsive Personality Disorder
301.9 Personality Disorder NOS

OTHER CONDITIONS THAT MAY BE A FOCUS OF CLINICAL ATTENTION

Psychological Factors Affecting Medical Condition

316 *Choose name based on nature of factors:*
　Mental Disorder Affecting Medical Condition
　Psychological Symptoms Affecting Medical Condition
　Personality Traits or Coping Style Affecting Medical Condition
　Maladaptive Health Behaviors Affecting Medical Condition
　Stress-Related Physiological Response Affecting Medical Condition
　Other or Unspecified Psychological Factors Affecting Medical Condition

Medication-Induced Movement Disorders

332.1 Neuroleptic-Induced Parkinsonism
333.92 Neuroleptic Malignant Syndrome
333.7 Neuroleptic-Induced Acute Dystonia
333.99 Neuroleptic-Induced Acute Akathisia
333.82 Neuroleptic-Induced Tardive Dyskinesia
333.1 Medication-Induced Postural Tremor
333.90 Medication-Induced Movement Disorder NOS

Other Medication-Induced Disorder

995.2 Adverse Effects of Medication NOS

Relational Problems

V61.9 Relational Problem Related to a Mental Disorder or General Medical Condition
V61.20 Parent-Child Relational Problem

V61.10 Partner Relational Problem
V61.8 Sibling Relational Problem
V62.81 Relational Problem NOS
Problems Related to Abuse or Neglect
V61.21 Physical Abuse of Child
V61.21 Sexual Abuse of Child
V61.21 Neglect of Child
——.— Physical Abuse of Adult
V61.12 (if by partner)
V62.83 (if by person other than partner)
——.— Sexual Abuse of Adult
V61.12 (if by partner)
V62.83 (if by person other than partner)
Additional Conditions That May Be a Focus of Clinical Attention
V15.81 Noncompliance with Treatment
V65.2 Malingering
V71.01 Adult Antisocial Behavior
V71.02 Childhood or Adolescent Antisocial Behavior
V62.89 Borderline Intellectual Functioning (coded on Axis II)
780.9 Age-Related Cognitive Decline
V62.82 Bereavement
V62.3 Academic Problem
V62.2 Occupational Problem
313.82 Identity Problem
V62.89 Religious or Spiritual Problem
V62.4 Acculturation Problem
V62.89 Phase of Life Problem

ADDITIONAL CODES
300.9 Unspecified Mental Disorder (nonpsychotic)
V71.09 No Diagnosis or Condition on Axis I
799.9 Diagnosis or Condition Deferred on Axis I
V71.09 No Diagnosis on Axis II
799.9 Diagnosis Deferred on Axis II

Assigning Nursing Diagnoses (NANDA) to Client Behaviors

Following is a list of client behaviors and the NANDA nursing diagnoses that correspond to the behaviors and that may be used in planning care for the client exhibiting the specific behavioral symptoms.

Behaviors	NANDA Nursing Diagnoses
Aggression; hostility	Risk for injury; Risk for other-directed violence
Anorexia or refusal to eat	Imbalanced nutrition: Less than body requirements
Anxious behavior	Anxiety (specify level)
Confusion; memory loss	Confusion, acute/chronic; Disturbed thought processes
Delusions	Disturbed thought processes
Denial of problems	Ineffective denial
Depressed mood or anger turned inward	Dysfunctional grieving
Detoxification; withdrawal from substances	Risk for injury
Difficulty making important life decision	Decisional conflict (specify)
Difficulty with interpersonal relationships	Impaired social interaction
Disruption in capability to perform usual responsibilities	Ineffective role performance
Dissociative behaviors (depersonalization; derealization)	Disturbed sensory perception (kinesthetic)
Expresses feelings of disgust about body or body part	Disturbed body image
Expresses lack of control over personal situation	Powerlessness
Flashbacks, nightmares, obsession with traumatic experience	Posttrauma syndrome

Behaviors	NANDA Nursing Diagnoses
Hallucinations	Disturbed sensory perception (auditory; visual)
Highly critical of self or others	Low self-esteem (chronic; situational)
HIV positive; altered immunity	Ineffective protection
Inability to meet basic needs	Self-care deficit (feeding; bathing/hygiene; dressing/grooming; toileting)
Insomnia or hypersomnia	Disturbed sleep pattern
Loose associations or flight of ideas	Impaired verbal communication
Manic hyperactivity	Risk for injury
Manipulative behavior	Ineffective coping
Multiple personalities; gender identity disturbance	Disturbed personal identity
Orgasm, problems with; lack of sexual desire	Sexual dysfunction
Overeating, compulsive	Risk for imbalanced nutrition: More than body requirements
Phobias	Fear
Physical symptoms as coping behavior	Ineffective coping
Projection of blame; rationalization of failures; denial of personal responsibility	Defensive coping
Ritualistic behaviors	Anxiety (severe); Ineffective coping
Seductive remarks; inappropriate sexual behaviors	Impaired social interaction
Self-mutilative behaviors	Self-mutilation; Risk for self-mutilation
Sexual behaviors (difficulty, limitations, or changes in; reported dissatisfaction)	Ineffective sexuality patterns

(Continued on following page)

(Continued)

Behaviors	NANDA Nursing Diagnoses
Stress from caring for chronically ill person	Caregiver role strain
Stress from locating to new environment	Relocation stress syndrome
Substance use as a coping-behavior	Ineffective coping
Substance use (denies use is a problem)	Ineffective denial
Suicidal	Risk for suicide; Risk for self-directed violence
Suspiciousness	Disturbed thought processes; Ineffective coping
Vomiting, excessive, self induced	Risk for deficient fluid volume
Withdrawn behavior	Social isolation

(Used with permission from Townsend, 3/e, 2005)

Psychiatric Terminology

A

abreaction. "Remembering with feeling"; bringing into conscious awareness painful events that have been repressed, and reexperiencing the emotions that were associated with the events.

adjustment disorder. A maladaptive reaction to an identifiable psychosocial stressor that occurs within 3 months after onset of the stressor. The individual shows impairment in social and occupational functioning or exhibits symptoms that are in excess of a normal and expectable reaction to the stressor.

affect. The behavioral expression of emotion; may be appropriate (congruent with the situation); inappropriate (incongruent with the situation); constricted or blunted (diminished range and intensity); or flat (absence of emotional expression).

agoraphobia. The fear of being in places or situations from which escape might be difficult (or embarrassing) or in which help might not be available in the event of a panic attack.

akathisia. Restlessness; an urgent need for movement. A type of extrapyramidal side effect associated with some antipsychotic medications.

akinesia. Muscular weakness or a loss or partial loss of muscle movement; a type of extrapyramidal side effect associated with some antipsychotic medications.

amnesia. An inability to recall important personal information that is too extensive to be explained by ordinary forgetfulness.

anhedonia. The inability to experience or even imagine any pleasant emotion.

anorexia. Loss of appetite.

anorgasmia. Inability to achieve orgasm.

anticipatory grief. A subjective state of emotional, physical, and social responses to an anticipated loss of a valued entity. The grief response is repeated once the loss actually occurs, but it may not be as intense as it might have been if anticipatory grieving had not occurred.

antisocial personality disorder. A pattern of socially irresponsible, exploitative, and guiltless behavior, evident in the tendency to fail to conform to the law, develop stable relationships, or sustain consistent employment; exploitation and manipulation of others for personal gain is common.

anxiety. Vague diffuse apprehension that is associated with feelings of uncertainty and helplessness.

associative looseness. Sometimes called loose associations, a thinking process characterized by speech in which ideas shift from one unrelated subject to another. The individual is unaware that the topics are unconnected.

ataxia. Muscular incoordination.

attitude. A frame of reference around which an individual organizes knowledge about his or her world. It includes an emotional element and can have a positive or negative connotation.

autism. A focus inward on a fantasy world and distorting or excluding the external environment; common in schizophrenia.

autistic disorder. The withdrawal of an infant or child into the self and into a fantasy world of his or her own creation. There is marked impairment in interpersonal functioning and communication and in imaginative play. Activities and interests are restricted and may be considered somewhat bizarre.

B

behavior modification. A treatment modality aimed at changing undesirable behaviors, using a system of reinforcement to bring about the modifications desired.

belief. An idea that one believes to be true. It can be rational, irrational, taken on faith, or a stereotypical idea.

bereavement overload. An accumulation of grief that occurs when an individual experiences many losses over a short period and is unable to resolve one before another is experienced. This phenomenon is common among the elderly.

bipolar disorder. Characterized by mood swings from profound depression to extreme euphoria (mania), with intervening periods of normalcy. Psychotic symptoms may or may not be present.

borderline personality disorder. A disorder characterized by a pattern of intense and chaotic relationships, with affective instability, fluctuating and extreme attitudes regarding other people, impulsivity, direct and indirect self-destructive behavior, and lack of a clear or certain sense of identity, life plan, or values.

boundaries. The level of participation and interaction between individuals and between subsystems. Boundaries denote physical and psychological space individuals identify as their own. They are sometimes referred to as limits.

C

catatonia. A type of schizophrenia that is typified by stupor or excitement: stupor characterized by extreme psychomotor retardation, mutism, negativism, and posturing; excitement by psychomotor agitation, in which the movements are frenzied and purposeless.

circumstantiality. In speaking, the delay of an individual to reach the point of a communication, owing to unnecessary and tedious details.

clang associations. A pattern of speech in which the choice of words is governed by sounds. Clang associations often take the form of rhyming.

codependency. An exaggerated dependent pattern of learned behaviors, beliefs, and feelings that make life painful. It is a dependence on people and things outside the self, along with neglect of the self to the point of having little self-identity.

cognition. Mental operations that relate to logic, awareness, intellect, memory, language, and reasoning powers.

cognitive therapy. A type of therapy in which the individual is taught to control thought distortions that are considered to be a factor in the development and maintenance of emotional disorders.

compensation. Covering up a real or perceived weakness by emphasizing a trait one considers more desirable.

concrete thinking. Thought processes that are focused on specifics rather than on generalities and immediate issues rather than eventual outcomes. Individuals who are experiencing concrete thinking are unable to comprehend abstract terminology.

confidentiality. The right of an individual to the assurance that his or her case will not be discussed outside the boundaries of the healthcare team.

crisis. Psychological disequilibrium in a person who confronts a hazardous circumstance that constitutes an important problem, which for the time he or she can neither escape nor solve with usual problem-solving resources.

crisis intervention. An emergency type of assistance in which the intervener becomes a part of the individual's life situation. The focus is to provide guidance and support to help mobilize the resources needed to resolve the crisis and restore or generate an improvement in previous level of functioning. Usually lasts no longer than 6 to 8 weeks.

culture. A particular society's entire way of living, encompassing shared patterns of belief, feeling, and knowledge that guide people's conduct and are passed down from generation to generation.

curandera. A female folk healer in the Latino culture.

curandero. A male folk healer in the Latino culture.

cycle of battering. Three phases of predictable behaviors that are repeated over time in a relationship between a batterer and a victim: tension-building phase; the acute battering incident; and the calm, loving respite (honeymoon) phase.

cyclothymia. A chronic mood disturbance involving numerous episodes of hypomania and depressed mood, of insufficient severity or duration to meet the criteria for bipolar disorder.

D

delayed grief. Also called *inhibited grief*. The absence of evidence of grief when it ordinarily would be expected.

delirium. A state of mental confusion and excitement characterized by disorientation for time and place, often with hallucinations, incoherent speech, and a continual state of aimless physical activity.

delusions. False personal beliefs, not consistent with a person's intelligence or cultural background. The individual continues to have the belief in spite of obvious proof that it is false and/or irrational.

dementia. Global impairment of cognitive functioning that is progressive and interferes with social and occupational abilities.

denial. Refusal to acknowledge the existence of a real situation and/or the feelings associated with it.

depersonalization. An alteration in the perception or experience of the self so that the feeling of one's own reality is temporarily lost.

derealization. An alteration in the experience or experience of the external world so that it seems strange or unreal.

Diagnostic and Statistical Manual of Mental Disorders, 4th edition, Text Revision (DSM-IV-TR). Standard nomenclature of emotional illness published by the American Psychiatric Association (APA) and used by all healthcare practitioners. It classifies mental illness and presents guidelines and diagnostic criteria for various mental disorders.

displacement. Feelings are transferred from one target to another that is considered less threatening or neutral.

double-bind communication. Communication described as contradictory that places an individual in a "double bind." It occurs when a statement is made and succeeded by a contradictory statement or when a statement is made accompanied by nonverbal expression that is inconsistent with the verbal communication.

dyspareunia. Pain during sexual intercourse.

dysthymia. A depressive neurosis. The symptoms are similar to, if somewhat milder than, those ascribed to major depression. There is no loss of contact with reality.

dystonia. Involuntary muscular movements (spasms) of the face, arms, legs, and neck; may occur as an extrapyramidal side effect of some antipsychotic medications.

E

echolalia. The parrot-like repetition, by an individual with loose ego boundaries, of the words spoken by another.

ego. One of the three elements of the personality identified by Freud as the rational self or "reality principle." The ego seeks to maintain harmony between the external world, the id, and the superego.

electroconvulsive therapy (ECT). A type of somatic treatment in which electric current is applied to the brain through electrodes placed on the temples. A grand mal seizure produces the desired effect. This is used with severely depressed patients refractory to antidepressant medications.

empathy. The ability to see beyond outward behavior and sense accurately another's inner experiencing. With empathy, one can accurately perceive and understand the meaning and relevance in the thoughts and feelings of another.

enmeshment. Exaggerated connectedness among family members. It occurs in response to diffuse boundaries in which there is overinvestment, overinvolvement, and lack of differentiation between individuals or subsystems.

ethnicity. The concept of people identifying with each other because of a shared heritage.

exhibitionism. A paraphilic disorder characterized by a recurrent urge to expose one's genitals to a stranger.

extrapyramidal symptoms (EPS). A variety of responses that originate outside the pyramidal tracts and in the basal ganglion of the brain. Symptoms may include tremors, chorea, dystonia, akinesia, and akathisia, and others may occur as a side effect of some antipsychotic medications.

F

family system. A system in which the parts of the whole may be the marital dyad, parent-child dyad, or sibling groups. Each of these subsystems is further divided into subsystems of individuals.

family therapy. A type of therapy in which the focus is on relationships within the family. The family is viewed as a system in which the members are interdependent, and a change in one creates change in all.

fight or flight. A syndrome of physical symptoms that result from an individual's real or perceived perception that harm or danger is imminent.

free association. A technique used to help individuals bring to consciousness material that has been repressed. The individual is encouraged to verbalize whatever comes into his or her mind, drifting naturally from one thought to another.

G

gains. The reinforcements an individual receives for somaticizing.

gender identity disorder. A sense of discomfort associated with an incongruence between biologically assigned gender and subjectively experienced gender.

generalized anxiety disorder. A disorder characterized by chronic (at least 6 months), unrealistic, and excessive anxiety and worry.

genogram. A graphic representation of a family system. It may cover several generations. Emphasis is on family roles and emotional relatedness among members. Genograms facilitate recognition of areas requiring change.

grief. A subjective state of emotional, physical, and social responses to the real or perceived loss of a valued entity. Change and failure can also be perceived as losses. The grief response consists of a set of relatively predictable behaviors that describe the subjective state that accompanies mourning.

group therapy. A therapy group, founded in a specific theoretical framework, led by a person with an advanced degree in psychology, social work, nursing, or medicine. The goal is to encourage improvement in interpersonal functioning.

H

hallucinations. False sensory perceptions not associated with real external stimuli. Hallucinations may involve any of the five senses.

histrionic personality disorder. Conscious or unconscious overly dramatic behavior used for drawing attention to oneself.

human immunodeficiency virus (HIV). The virus that is the etiological agent that produces the immunosuppression resulting in AIDS.

hypersomnia. Excessive sleepiness or seeking excessive amounts of sleep.

hypertensive crisis. A potentially life-threatening syndrome that results when an individual taking MAOIs eats a product high in tyramine or uses an SSRI too soon either before or after stopping an MAOI.

hypnosis. A treatment for disorders brought on by repressed anxiety. The individual is directed into a state of subconsciousness and assisted, through suggestions, to recall certain events that he or she cannot recall when conscious.

hypomania. A mild form of mania. Symptoms are excessive hyperactivity, but not severe enough to cause marked impairment in social or occupational functioning or to require hospitalization.

I

id. One of the three components of the personality identified by Freud as the "pleasure principle." The id is the locus of instinctual drives; is present at birth; and compels the infant to satisfy needs and seek immediate gratification.

illusion. A misperception of a real external stimulus.

incest. Sexual exploitation of a child under 18 years of age by a relative or nonrelative who holds a position of trust in the family.

integration. The process used with individuals with dissociative identity disorder in an effort to bring all the personalities together into one; usually achieved through hypnosis.

intellectualization. An attempt to avoid expressing actual emotions associated with a stressful situation by using the intellectual processes of logic, reasoning, and analysis.

introjection. The beliefs and values of another individual are internalized and symbolically become a part of the self to the extent that the feeling of separateness or distinctness is lost.

isolation. The separation of a thought or a memory from the feeling, tone, or emotions associated with it (sometimes called emotional isolation).

J

justice. An ethical principle reflecting that all individuals should be treated equally and fairly.

K

kleptomania. A recurrent failure to resist impulses to steal objects not needed for personal use or monetary value.

Korsakoff's psychosis. A syndrome of confusion, loss of recent memory, and confabulation in alcoholics, caused by a deficiency of thiamine. It often occurs together with Wernicke's encephalopathy and may be termed Wernicke-Korsakoff syndrome.

L

libido. Freud's term for the psychic energy used to fulfill basic physiological needs or instinctual drives such as hunger, thirst, and sexuality.

limbic system. The part of the brain that is sometimes called the "emotional brain." It is associated with feelings of fear and anxiety; anger and aggression; love, joy, and hope; and with sexuality and social behavior.

long-term memory. Memory for remote events, or those that occurred many years ago. The type of memory that is preserved in the elderly individual.

loss. The experience of separation from something of personal importance.

luto. The word for mourning in the Mexican-American culture that is symbolized by wearing black, black and white, or dark clothing and by subdued behavior.

M

magical thinking. A primitive form of thinking in which an individual believes that thinking about a possible occurrence can make it happen.

mania. A type of bipolar disorder in which the predominant mood is elevated, expansive, or irritable. Motor activity is frenzied and excessive. Psychotic features may or may not be present.

melancholia. A severe form of major depressive episode. Symptoms are exaggerated, and interest or pleasure in virtually all activities is lost.

mental imagery. A method of stress reduction that employs the imagination. The individual focuses imagination on a scenario that is particularly relaxing to him or her (e.g., a scene on a quiet seashore, a mountain atmosphere, or floating through the air on a fluffy white cloud).

milieu therapy. Also called therapeutic community, or therapeutic environment, this type of therapy consists of a scientific structuring of the environment in order to effect behavioral changes and to improve the individual's psychological health and functioning.

modeling. Learning new behaviors by imitating the behaviors of others.

mood. An individual's sustained emotional tone, which significantly influences behavior, personality, and perception.

mourning. The psychological process (or stages) through which the individual passes on the way to successful adaptation to the loss of a valued object.

N

narcissistic personality disorder. A disorder characterized by an exaggerated sense of self-worth. These individuals lack empathy and are hypersensitive to the evaluation of others.

neologism. New words that an individual invents that are meaningless to others but have symbolic meaning to the psychotic person.

neuroleptic. Antipsychotic medication used to prevent or control psychotic symptoms.

neuroleptic malignant syndrome (NMS). A rare but potentially fatal complication of treatment with neuroleptic drugs. Symptoms include severe muscle rigidity, high fever, tachycardia, fluctuations in blood pressure, diaphoresis, and rapid deterioration of mental status to stupor and coma.

neurotransmitter. A chemical that is stored in the axon terminals of the presynaptic neuron. An electrical impulse through the neuron stimulates the release of the neurotransmitter into the synaptic cleft, which in turn determines whether another electrical impulse is generated.

nursing diagnosis. A clinical judgment about individual, family, or community responses to actual and potential health problems/processes. Nursing diagnoses provide the basis for selection of nursing interventions to achieve outcomes for which the nurse is accountable.

nursing process. A dynamic, systematic process by which nurses assess, diagnose, identify outcomes, plan, implement, and evaluate nursing care. It has been called "nursing's scientific methodology." Nursing process gives order and consistency to nursing intervention.

O

obesity. The state of having a body mass index of 30 or above.

object constancy. The phase in the separation/individuation process when the child learns to relate to objects in an effective, constant manner. A sense of separateness is established, and the child is able to internalize a sustained image of the loved object or person when out of sight.

obsessive-compulsive disorder. Recurrent thoughts or ideas (obsessions) that an individual is unable to put out of his or her mind, and actions that an individual is unable to refrain from performing (compulsions). The obsessions and compulsions are severe enough to interfere with social and occupational functioning.

oculogyric crisis. An attack of involuntary deviation and fixation of the eyeballs, usually in the upward position. It may last for several minutes or hours and may occur as an extrapyramidal side effect of some antipsychotic medications.

P

panic disorder. A disorder characterized by recurrent panic attacks, the onset of which is unpredictable, and manifested by intense apprehension, fear, or terror, often associated with feelings of impending doom and accompanied by intense physical discomfort.

paranoia. A term that implies extreme suspiciousness. Paranoid schizophrenia is characterized by persecutory delusions and hallucinations of a threatening nature.

passive-aggressive behavior. Behavior that defends an individual's own basic rights by expressing resistance to social and occupational demands. Sometimes called indirect aggression, this behavior takes the form of sly, devious, and undermining actions that express the opposite of what the person is really feeling.

pedophilia. Recurrent urges and sexually arousing fantasies involving sexual activity with a prepubescent child.

perseveration. Persistent repetition of the same word or idea in response to different questions.

personality. Deeply ingrained patterns of behavior, which include the way one relates to, perceives, and thinks about the environment and oneself.

phobia. An irrational fear.

phobia, social. The fear of being humiliated in social situations.

postpartum depression. Depression that occurs during the postpartum period. It may be related to hormonal changes, tryptophan metabolism, or alterations in membrane transport during the early postpartum period. Other predisposing factors may also be influential.

posttraumatic stress disorder (PTSD). A syndrome of symptoms that develop following a psychologically distressing event that is outside the range of usual human experience (e.g., rape, war). The individual is unable to put the experience out of his or her mind and has nightmares, flashbacks, and panic attacks.

preassaultive tension state. Behaviors predictive of potential violence. They include excessive motor activity, tense posture, defiant affect, clenched teeth and fists, and other arguing, demanding, and threatening behaviors.

priapism. Prolonged painful penile erection, may occur as an adverse effect of some antidepressant medications, particularly trazodone.

progressive relaxation. A method of deep muscle relaxation in which each muscle group is alternately tensed and relaxed in a systematic order with the person concentrating on the contrast of sensations experienced from tensing and relaxing.

projection. Attributing to another person feelings or impulses unacceptable to oneself.

pseudodementia. Symptoms of depression that mimic those of dementia.

psychomotor retardation. Extreme slowdown of physical movements. Posture slumps; speech is slowed; digestion becomes sluggish. Common in severe depression.

psychotic disorder. A serious psychiatric disorder in which there is a gross disorganization of the personality, a marked disturbance in reality testing, and the impairment of interpersonal functioning and relationship to the external world.

R

rape. The expression of power and dominance by means of sexual violence, most commonly by men over women, although men may also be rape victims. Rape is considered an act of aggression, not of passion.

rapport. The development between two people in a relationship of special feelings based on mutual acceptance, warmth, friendliness, common interest, a sense of trust, and a nonjudgmental attitude.

rationalization. Attempting to make excuses or formulate logical reasons to justify unacceptable feelings or behaviors.

reaction formation. Preventing unacceptable or undesirable thoughts or behaviors from being expressed by exaggerating opposite thoughts or types of behaviors.

reframing. Changing the conceptual or emotional setting or viewpoint in relation to which a situation is experienced and placing it in another frame that fits the "facts" of the same concrete situation equally well or even better and thereby changing its entire meaning.

regression. A retreat to an earlier level of development and the comfort measures associated with that level of functioning.

reminiscence therapy. A process of life review by elderly individuals that promotes self-esteem and provides assistance in working through unresolved conflicts from the past.

repression. The involuntary blocking of unpleasant feelings and experiences from one's awareness.

ritualistic behavior. Purposeless activities that an individual performs repeatedly in an effort to decrease anxiety (e.g., handwashing); common in obsessive-compulsive disorder.

S

schizoid personality disorder. A profound defect in the ability to form personal relationships or to respond to others in any meaningful, emotional way.

schizotypal personality disorder. A disorder characterized by odd and eccentric behavior, not decompensating to the level of schizophrenia.

self-esteem. The amount of regard or respect that individuals have for themselves. It is a measure of worth that they place on their abilities and judgments.

shaman. The Native American "medicine man" or folk healer.

shaping. In learning, one shapes the behavior of another by giving reinforcements for increasingly closer approximations to the desired behavior.

short-term memory. The ability to remember events that occurred very recently. This ability deteriorates with age.

social skills training. Educational opportunities through role-play for the person with schizophrenia to learn appropriate social interaction skills and functional skills that are relevant to daily living.

splitting. A primitive ego defense mechanism in which the person is unable to integrate and accept both positive and negative feelings. In their view, people – including themselves – and life situations are all good or all bad. This trait is common in borderline personality disorder.

stereotyping. The process of classifying all individuals from the same culture or ethnic group as identical.

sublimation. The rechanneling of personal and/or socially unacceptable drives or impulses into activities that are tolerable and constructive.

substance abuse. Use of psychoactive drugs that poses significant hazards to health and interferes with social, occupational, psychological, or physical functioning.

substance dependence. Physical dependence is identified by the inability to stop using a substance despite attempts to do so; a continual use of the substance despite adverse consequences; a developing tolerance; and the development of withdrawal symptoms upon cessation or decreased intake. Psychological dependence is said to exist when a substance is perceived by the user to be necessary to maintain an optimal state of personal well-being, interpersonal relations, or skill performance.

substitution therapy. The use of various medications to decrease the intensity of symptoms in an individual who is withdrawing from, or experiencing the effects of excessive use of, substances.

superego. One of the three elements of the personality identified by Freud that represents the conscience and the culturally determined restrictions that are placed on an individual.

suppression. The voluntary blocking from one's awareness of unpleasant feelings and experiences.

symbiotic relationship. A type of "psychic fusion" that occurs between two people; it is unhealthy in that severe anxiety is generated in one or both if separation is indicated. A symbiotic relationship is normal between infant and mother.

sympathy. The actual sharing of another's thoughts and behaviors. Differs from empathy, in that with empathy one experiences an objective understanding of what another is feeling, rather than actually sharing those feelings.

systematic desensitization. A treatment for phobias in which the individual is taught to relax and then asked to imagine various components of the phobic stimulus on a graded hierarchy, moving from that which produces the least fear to that which produces the most.

T

tangentiality. The inability to get to the point of a story. The speaker introduces many unrelated topics, until the original topic of discussion is lost.

tardive dyskinesia. Syndrome of symptoms characterized by bizarre facial and tongue movements, a stiff neck, and difficulty swallowing. It may occur as an adverse effect of long-term therapy with some antipsychotic medications.

thought-stopping technique. A self-taught technique that an individual uses each time he or she wishes to eliminate intrusive or negative, unwanted thoughts from awareness.

triangles. A three-person emotional configuration, which is considered the basic building block of the family system. When anxiety becomes too great between two family members, a third person is brought in to form a triangle. Triangles are dysfunctional in that they offer relief from anxiety through diversion rather than through resolution of the issue.

trichotillomania. The recurrent failure to resist impulses to pull out one's own hair.

tyramine. An amino acid found in aged cheeses or other aged, overripe, and fermented foods; broad beans; pickled herring; beef or chicken liver; preserved meats; beer and wine; yeast products; chocolate; caffeinated drinks; canned figs; sour cream; yogurt; soy sauce; and some over-the-counter cold medications and diet pills. If foods high in tyramine content are consumed when an individual is taking MAOIs, a potentially life-threatening syndrome called hypertensive crisis can result.

U

unconditional positive regard. Carl Rogers' term for the respect and dignity of an individual regardless of his or her unacceptable behavior.

undoing. A mechanism used to symbolically negate or cancel out a previous action or experience that one finds intolerable.

universality. One curative factor of groups (identified by Yalom) in which individuals realize that they are not alone in a problem and in the thoughts and feelings they are experiencing. Anxiety is relieved by the support and understanding of others in the group who share similar experiences.

V

values. Personal beliefs about the truth, beauty, or worth of a thought, object, or behavior that influences an individual's actions.

velorio. In the Mexican-American culture, following a death, large numbers of family and friends gather for a *velorio*, a festive watch over the body of the deceased person before burial.

W

Wernicke's encephalopathy. A brain disorder caused by thiamine deficiency and characterized by visual disturbances, ataxia, somnolence, stupor, and, without thiamine replacement, death.

word salad. A group of words that are put together in a random fashion without any logical connection.

References

Aiken T. Legal, Ethical and Political Issues in Nursing, 2nd ed. Philadelphia: FA Davis, 2004

American Hospital Association. A Patient's Bill of Rights. Accessed 1/24/04 at: http://joann980.tripod.com/myhomeontheweb/id20.html

American Psychiatric Association. Diagnostic and Statistical Manual of Mental Disorders, 4th ed., Text Revision. Washington, DC: American Psychiatric Association, 2000

American Psychiatric Nurses Association (APNA). APNA Position Statement on Seclusion and Restraint. Accessed 1/24/2004 at: www.apna.org/resources/positionpapers.html

Antai-Otong D. Psychiatric Nursing: Biological and Behavioral Concepts. Clifton Park, NY: Thomson Delmar Learning, 2003

Anton RF et al. Comparison of Bio-Rad %CDT TIA and CDTect as Laboratory Markers of Heavy Alcohol Use and Their Relationships with γ-Glutamyl transferase. Clinical Chemistry 2001; 47(10): 1769–1775

APA 2000 Gender Advisory Panel: Terms of Reference. Accessed 7/17/04 at: www.who.int/reproductive-health/pcc2001/documents/gaptorrev01.doc

Arana GW, Rosenbaum JF. Handbook of Psychiatric Drug Therapy, 4th ed. Philadelphia: Lippincott Williams & Wilkins, 2000

Aripiprazole. Mosby's Drug Consult. Accessed 8/1/04 at: http://www.mosbysdrugconsult.com/DrugConsult/003577.html

Autonomic nervous system. Table 1: Responses of major organs to autonomic nerve impulses. Update in Anaesthesia 1995; issue 5, article 6. Accessed 1/24/04 at: http://www.nda.ox.ac.uk/wfsa/html/u05/u05_b02.htm

Bateson G. Steps to an Ecology of Mind. London: Paladin, 1973

Bateson G. Mind and Nature: A Necessary Unity. London: Wildwood House, 1979

Bleuler E. Dementia Praecox or the Group of Schizophrenias (Zinkin J, Trans). New York: International University Press, 1911

Boszormenyi-Nagy I, Krasner BR. Between Give and Take: A Clinical Guide to Contextual Therapy. New York: Brunner/Mazel, 1986

Bowen M. Family Therapy in Clinical Practice. New Jersey: Aronson, 1994

Brigham and Women's Hospital. Depression. A Guide to Diagnosis and Treatment. Boston, MA: Brigham and Women's Hospital, 2001:9

Bromet EJ, Dew MA, Eaton W. Epidemiology of psychosis with special reference to schizophrenia. In: Tsuang MT, Tohen M, Zahner GEP, eds. Textbook in Psychiatric Epidemiology. New York: Wiley-Liss, 1995:283–300

Brown GW, Birley JL, Wing JK. Influence of family life on the course of schizophrenic disorders: A replication. Br J Psychiatry 1972; 121(562):241–258

Brown AS, Susser ES. Epidemiology of schizophrenia: Findings implicate neurodevelopmental insults early in life. In: Kaufman CA, Gorman JM, eds. Schizophrenia: New Directions for Clinical Research and Treatment. Larchmont, NY: Mary Ann Liebert, Inc., 1996:105–119

Burgess AW, Hartman CR. Rape trauma and posttraumatic stress disorder. In: McBride AB, Austin JK, eds. Psychiatric Mental Health Nursing: Integrating the Behavioral and Biological Sciences. Philadelphia: WB Saunders, 1996:53–81

Buse JB, Cavazzoni P, Hornbuckle K, Hutchins D, Breier A, Jovanovic L. A retrospective cohort study of diabetes mellitus and antipsychotic treatment in the United States. J Clin Epidemiol 2003; 56:164–170

Chenitz WC, Stone JT, Salisbury SA. Clinical Gerontological Nursing: A Guide to Advanced Practice. Philadelphia: WB Saunders, 1991

Child Abuse Prevention Treatment Act, originally enacted in 1974 (PL 93–247), 42 USC 5101 et seq; 42 USC 5116 et seq. Accessed 9/25/04 at: http://www.acf.hhs.gov/programs/cb/laws/capta/

Christianson JR, Blake RH. The grooming process in father-daughter incest. In: Horton A, Johnson BL, Roundy LM,

Williams D, eds. The Incest Perpetrator: A Family Member No One Wants to Treat. Newbury Park, CA: Sage, 1990:88–98

Cruz M, Pincus HA. Research on the Influence that Communication in Psychiatric Encounters Has on Treatment. Psychiatr Serv 2002; 53:1253–1265

Cycle of Violence. Accessed 8/7/04 at: http://www.ojp.usdoj.gov/ovc/help/cycle.htm

Davies T. Psychosocial factors and relapse of schizophrenia [Editorial]. BMJ 1994; 309:353–354

Deglin JH, Vallerand AH. Davis's Drug Guide for Nurses, 9th ed. Philadelphia: FA Davis, 2005

ECNP: Zyprexa (Olanzapine) Superior to Depakote (Valproate) for Acute Mania in Bipolar Disorder. Accessed 8/1/04 at: http://www.pslgroup.com/dg/1E0626.htm

Emergency Commitments: Psychiatric emergencies. Accessed 1/24/04 at: http://www.pinofpa.org/resources/fact-12.html

Ewing JA. Detecting alcoholism: The CAGE Questionnaire. JAMA 1984; 252:1905–1907

Faraone S. Prevalence of adult ADHD in the US [Abstract]. Presented at American Psychiatric Association, May 6, 2004. Accessed 9/24/04 at: http://www.pslgroup.com/dg/2441a2.htm

Folstein M, Folstein SG, McHugh P. Mini-Mental State, a practical method for grading the cognitive state of patients for the clinician. J Psychiatr Res 1975; 12:189–198

Frazer A, Molinoff P, Winokur A. Biological Bases of Brain Function and Disease. New York: Raven Press, 1994

Freeman A, Pretzer J, Fleming B, Simon KM. Clinical Applications of Cognitive Therapy. New York: Plenum Press, 1990

Fuller MA, Sajatovic M: Drug Information Handbook for Psychiatry, 2nd ed. Cleveland: Lexi-Comp, 2000

Ghaemi SN, Hsu DJ, Soldami F, Goodwin FK. Antidepressants in bipolar disorder: The case for caution. Bipolar Disord 2003; 5(6):421–433

Goroll AH, Mulley AG Jr. Primary Care Medicine, 4th ed. Philadelphia: Lippincott Williams & Wilkins, 1995

Guy W, ed. ECDEU Assessment Manual for Psychopharmacology. (DHEW Publ. No. 76–338), Rev. ed. Washington, DC: US Department of Health, Education and Welfare, 1976.

Health Canada: Important Drug Safety Information for Paroxetine. Accessed 9/25/04 at: http://www.hc-sc.gc.ca/hpfb-dgpsa/tpd-dpt/paxil_hpc_e.html

Health Insurance Portability and Accountability Act (HIPAA). Accessed 1/18/04 at: http://www.ihs.gov/AdminMngrResources/HIPAA/index.cfm

Holkup P. Evidence-Based Protocol. Elderly Suicide: Secondary Prevention. Iowa City: University of Iowa Gerontological Nursing Interventions Research Center, Research Dissemination Core, June 2002:56

Hunt M. The Story of Psychology. New York: Anchor Books, 1994

International Society of Psychiatric–Mental Health Nurses (ISPN). ISPN Position Statement on the Use of Seclusion and Restraint (November 1999). Accessed 10/1/04 at: http://www.ispn-psych.org

Jahoda M. Current Concepts of Positive Mental Health. New York: Basic Books, 1958

Johnson TB. National Association of School Psychologists Communiqué. October 2003; vol. 32, No. 2. Accessed 9/25/2004 at: http://www.nasponline.org/publications/cq322depressionwarnings.html

Joint Commission on Accreditation of Healthcare Organizations (JCAHO): Restraint and Seclusion. Accessed 1/18/04 at: http://www.jcaho.org/

Kansas Child Abuse Prevention Council (KCAPC). A Guide about Child Abuse and Neglect. Wichita, KS: National Committee for Prevention of Child Abuse and Parents Anonymous, 1992

Kaplan HI, Sadock BJ. Comprehensive Textbook of Psychiatry, 5th ed. Baltimore: Williams & Wilkins, 1989

Keck PE Jr. Evaluating treatment decisions in bipolar depression. MedScape July 30, 2003. Accessed 7/3/04 at http:www.medscape.com/viewprogram/2571

Kerr ME, Bowen M. Family Evaluation. New York: WW Norton, 1988

Kessler RC, McGonagle KA, Zhao S, et al. Lifetime and 12-month prevalence of DSM-III-R psychiatric disorders in the United States. Results from the National Comorbidity Survey. Arch Gen Psychiatry 1994; 51:8–19.

Krupnick SLW. Psychopharmacology. In Lego S (ed). Psychiatric Nursing: A Comprehensive Reference, 2nd ed. Philadelphia: Lippincott-Raven, 1996: 499–541

Kübler-Ross E. On Death and Dying. New York: Touchstone 1997

Kukull WA, Bowen JD. Dementia Epidemiology. Med Clin North Am 2002; 86:3

Laben JK, Crofts Yorker B. Legal issues in advanced practice psychiatric nursing. In Burgess AW, ed. Advanced Practice Psychiatric Nursing. Stamford, CT: Appleton & Lange, 1998:101–118

Lego S. Psychiatric Nursing. A Comprehensive Reference, 2nd ed. Philadelphia: Lippincott-Raven 1996

Linehan MM. Cognitive-Behavioral Treatment of Borderline Personality Disorder. New York: Guilford Press, 1993

Lippitt R, White RK. An experimental study of leadership and group life. In Maccoby EE, Newcomb TM, Hartley EL, eds. Readings in Social Psychology, 3rd ed. New York: Holt Rinehart & Winston, 1958

Lubman DI, Castle DJ. Late-onset schizophrenia: Make the right diagnosis when psychosis emerges after age 60. Curr Psychiatry Online 2002; 1(12). Accessed 8/7/04 at: http://www.currentpsychiatry.com/2002_12/1202_schizo.asp

M'Naughton Rule. Psychiatric News April 19, 2002; 37(8)

Major Theories of Family Therapy. Accessed 8/2/04 at: http://www.goldentriadfilms.com/films/theory.htm

Maxmen JS, Ward NG. Psychotropic Drugs Fast Facts, 2nd ed. New York: WW Norton, 1995

McGoldrick M, Giordano J, Pearce JK. Ethnicity and Family Therapy, 2nd ed. New York: Guilford Press, 1996

Meltzer HY, Baldessarini RJ. Reducing the risk for suicide in schizophrenia and affective disorders. Academic highlights. J Clin Psychiatry 2003; 64:9

Manos PJ. 10-Point clock test screens for cognitive impairment in clinic and hospital settings. Psychiatric Times October 1998; 15(10). Accessed 9/20/04 at: http://www.psychiatrictimes.com/p981049.html

Mini-Mental State Examination form. Available from Psychological Assessment Resources, Inc., 16204 North Florida Avenue, Lutz, Florida (see http://www.parinc.com/index.cfm)

Murray RB, Zentner JP. Health Assessment and Promotion Strategies through the Life Span, 6th ed. Stamford, CT: Appleton & Lange, 1997

Myers E. LPNNotes. Philadelphia: FA Davis, 2004

Myers E. RNotes. Philadelphia: FA Davis, 2003

Nagy Ledger of Merits. Accessed 8/2/04 at http://www.behavenet.com/capsules/treatment/famsys/ldgmrts.htm

Nonacs RM. Postpartum depression. eMedicine June 17, 2004. Accessed 7/17/04 at: http://www.emedicine.com/med/topic3408.htm

Olanzapine + VA, Lithium vs Valproic Acid, Lithium: Therapeutic Use: Bipolar Disorders Accessed 8/1/04 at http://www.luinst.org/cp/en/CNSforum/literature/trial_reports/reports/889317.html

Paquette M. Managing Anger Effectively. Accessed 8/2/04 at: http://www.nurseweek.com/ce/ce2904.html

Patient's Bill of Rights: American Hospital Association. Accessed 1/18/04 at: http://joann980.tripod.com/myhomeontheweb/id20.html

Peplau H. A working definition of anxiety. In: Bird S, Marshall M, eds. Some Clinical Approaches to Psychiatric Nursing. New York: Macmillan, 1963

Peplau HE. Interpersonal Relations in Nursing. New York: Springer, 1992

Poulin C, Webster I, Single E. Alcohol disorders in Canada as indicated by the CAGE Questionnaire. Can Med Assoc J 1997; 157(11):1529-1535

Rakel R: Saunders Manual of Medical Practice, 2nd ed. Philadelphia: WB Saunders, 2000

Reiger DA, Farmer ME, Rae D, Locke BZ, Keith SJ, Judd LL, Goodwin FK. Comorbidity of mental disorders with alcohol and other drug abuse. JAMA 1990; 246(19):2511–2518

Reno J. Domestic Violence Awareness. Office of the Attorney General. Accessed on 9/25/04 at: http://www.ojp.usdoj.gov/ovc/help/cycle.htm (last updated 4/19/2001)

Rupp A, Keith SJ: The costs of schizophrenia. Assessing the burden. Psychiatr Clin North Am 1993; 16(2):413–423

Satcher D. Mental Health: A Report of the Surgeon General. Rockville, MD: US Department of Health and Human Services, Substance Abuse and Mental Health Services Administration, Center for Mental Health Services, National Institutes of Health, National Institute of Mental Health, 1999. Accessed 1/19/04 at: http://www.surgeongeneral.gov/library/mentalhealth/home.html

Scanlon VC, Sanders T. Essentials of Anatomy and Physiology, 3rd ed. Philadelphia: FA Davis, 1999

Schloendorff v. Society of New York Hospital, 105 NE 92 (NY 1914)

Schnell ZB, Van Leeuwen AM, Kranpitz TR. Davis's Comprehensive Handbook of Laboratory and Diagnostic Tests with Nursing Implications. Philadelphia: FA Davis, 2003

Selye H. The Stress of Life. New York: McGraw-Hill, 1976

Selzer ML, Vinokur A, van Rooijen L. A self-administered Short Michigan Alcoholism Screening Test (SMAST). J Stud Alcohol 1975; 36:117–126

Sexual health. In: World Health Organization website. Accessed 7/17/04 at: http://www.who.int/reproductive-health/gender/sexual_health.html

Shader I. Approaches to the treatment of schizophrenia. In: Manual of Psychiatric Therapeutics. Boston: Little, Brown, 1994:311–336

Shapiro F. Eye Movement Desensitization and Reprocessing:

Basic Principles, Protocols, and Procedures. New York: Guilford Press, 1995

Shea CA, Pelletier LR, Poster EC, Stuart GW, Verhey MP, American Psychiatric Nurses Association. Advanced Practice Nursing in Psychiatric and Mental Health Care. St. Louis: CV Mosby, 1999

Sheikh JI, Yesavage JA. Geriatric Depression Scale (GDS): Recent evidence and development of a shorter version. In: Brink TL, ed. Clinical Gerontology: A Guide to Assessment and Intervention. New York: Haworth Press, 1986:165–173

Skinner K. The therapeutic milieu: Making it work. J Psychiatr Nursing Mental Health Serv 1979; 17:38–44

Sonne SC, Brady KT. Bipolar Disorder and Alcoholism. National Institute on Alcohol Abuse and Alcoholism (NIAAA). Posted November 2002. Accessed 7/3/04 at: http://www.niaaa.nih.gov/publications/arh26–2/103–108.htm

Stiles MM, Koren C, Walsh K. Identifying elder abuse in the primary care setting. Clin Geriatr 2002; 10(7). Accessed 8/7/04 at: www.mmhc.com

Stuart MR, Lieberman JA. The Fifteen Minute Hour: Applied Psychotherapy for the Primary Care Physician, 3rd ed. Westport, CT: Praeger, 1993:101–183

Suicide Risk Factors. Accessed 8/7/04 at: http://www.infoline.org/crisis/risk.asp

Tai B, Blaine J. Naltrexone: An Antagonist Therapy for Heroin Addiction. Presented at the National Institute on Drug Abuse, November 12–13, 1997. Accessed 7/3/2004 at: http://www.nida.nih.gov/MeetSum/naltrexone.html

Tarasoff v. Regents of University of California (17 Cal. 3d 425 – July 1, 1976. S. F. No. 23042)

Tasman A, Kay J, Lieberman JA. Psychiatry. Philadelphia: WB Saunders, 1997

Townsend MC. Essentials of Psychiatric Mental Health Nursing, 3rd ed. Philadelphia: FA Davis, 2005

Townsend MC. Psychiatric Mental Health Nursing: Concepts of Care, 4th ed. Philadelphia: FA Davis, 2003

Travelbee J. Interpersonal Aspects of Nursing. Philadelphia: FA Davis, 1971

Tucker K. Milan Approach to Family Therapy: A Critique. Accessed 8/2/04 at: http://www.priory.com/psych/milan.htm

US Public Health Services (USPHS). The Surgeon General's Call to Action to Prevent Suicide. Washington, DC: US Department of Health and Human Services, 1999. Accessed 1/18/04 at: http://www.surgeongeneral.gov/library/calltoaction/calltoaction.htm

Van der Kolk BA. Trauma and memory. In: Van der Kolk BA, McFarlane AC, Weisaeth L. Traumatic Stress. New York: Guilford Press, 1996

Virginia Satir. In Allyn & Bacon Family Therapy Website. Accessed 8/2/04 at: http://www.abacon.com/famtherapy/satir.html

Walker LE. The Battered Woman. New York: Harper & Row, 1979

Yalom ID. The Theory and Practice of Group Psychotherapy, 4th ed. New York: Basic Books, 1995

Yatham LN, Kusumakar V, Parikh SV, Haslam DR, Matte R, Sharma V, Kennedy S. Bipolar depression: treatment options. Can J Psychiatry 1997; 42(Suppl 2):87S-91S

Yesavage JA, Brink TL, Rose TL, Lum O, Huang V, Adey MB, Leirer VO. Development and validation of a geriatric depression screening scale: A preliminary report. J Psychiatr Res 1983; 17:37–49

Young People Advised Not to Use Seroxat. 10 Downing Street, Newsroom, October 6, 2003. Accessed 9/25/04 at: http://www.number-10.gov.uk/output/page3851.asp

Zyprexa (Eli Lilly Company). Accessed 8/1/04 at: http://pi.lilly.com/us/zyprexa-pi.pdf

PsychNotes

Credits

Dosage and drug data in Psychotropic DrugTab from Tables 21.2, p 293; 21.3, p 295; 21.6, p. 301; and 21.8, p. 304, in Townsend MC. Psychiatric Mental Health Nursing, 4th ed., 2003, and from Deglin JH, Vallerand AH: Davis's Drug Guide

Index

Note: Page numbers followed by f refer to figures/illustrations.